GETTING
a *Grip*
on
Diabetes

D0038901

Quick Tips & Techniques
for kids and teens

Spike Nasmyth Loy   Bo Nasmyth Loy

Janet Silverstein, MD and Marc Weigensberg, MD

Foreword by Diana Schwarzbein, MD, author of *The Schwarzbein Principle*

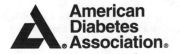

**American
Diabetes
Association**

Director, Book Publishing, John Fedor; *Editor*, Sherrye Landrum; *Production Manager*, Peggy M. Rote; *Composition*, Circle Graphics, Inc.; *Cover Design*, VC Graphics Design Studio; *Printer*, Port City Press, Inc.

Printed in the United States of America
3 5 7 9 10 8 6 4 2

The suggestions and information contained in this publication are generally consistent with the *Clinical Practice Recommendations* and other policies of the American Diabetes Association, but they do not represent the policy or position of the Association or any of its boards or committees. Reasonable steps have been taken to ensure the accuracy of the information presented. However, the American Diabetes Association cannot ensure the safety or efficacy of any product or service described in this publication. Individuals are advised to consult a physician or other appropriate health care professional before undertaking any diet or exercise program or taking any medication referred to in this publication. Professionals must use and apply their own professional judgment, experience, and training and should not rely solely on the information contained in this publication before prescribing any diet, exercise, or medication. The American Diabetes Association—its officers, directors, employees, volunteers, and members—assumes no responsibility or liability for personal or other injury, loss, or damage that may result from the suggestions or information in this publication.

⊗ The paper in this publication meets the requirements of the ANSI Standard Z39.48-1992 (permanence of paper).

ADA titles may be purchased for business or promotional use or for special sales. To purchase this book in large quantities, or for custom editions of this book with your logo, contact Lee Romano Sequeira, Special Sales & Promotions, at the address below, or at LRomano@diabetes.org or 703-299-2046.

American Diabetes Association
1701 North Beauregard Street
Alexandria, Virginia 22311

Library of Congress Cataloging-in-Publication Data

Loy, Spike Nasmyth, 1980-
     Getting a grip on diabetes: quick tips & techniques for kids and teens / Spike Nasmyth Loy, Bo Nasmyth Loy.
          p. cm.
     Includes index.
     ISBN 1-58040-053-1 (pbk. : alk. Paper)
     1. Diabetes in children—Juvenile literature. 2. Diabetes in children—Patients—Home care—Juvenile literature. 3. Diabetes in adolescence—Patients—Home care—Juvenile literature. [1. Diabetes. 2. Diseases.] I. Loy, Bo Nasmyth, 1982- II. Title.

RJ420.D5 L695 2000
618.92'462—dc21   00-050217

Contents

Foreword

These are exciting times! There are new advances being made in the field of medicine almost on a daily basis. Fetal islet cell transplant research is getting closer to being perfected, and nasal spray insulin may be just around the corner. For patients with type 1 diabetes, these breakthroughs could mean a life well lived without the need for injections! But since these advances are not available yet, it is important for the type 1 diabetic patients to learn how to take care of themselves in the meantime. And this is what this diabetes manual, written by Spike and Bodie Loy, helps you do. This manual shares all their helpful hints of what it takes to be prepared for every situation. It not only helps the patients with diabetes but their families as well.

Once the diagnosis of type 1 diabetes is made, the therapy can begin. I believe that five areas of life need to be addressed to treat diabetes completely. These are 1) stresses, 2) nutrition, 3) avoidance of chemicals and stimulants, 4) exercise, and 5) insulin therapy.

Insulin is a food-storing hormone and, therefore, is one of the most important growth hormones. It helps to balance blood levels of sugar by storing excess blood sugar into cells and helps to maintain the pH balance of the blood by storing amino acids and fatty acids into cells. There are five anti-insulin hormones: adrenaline, norepinephrine, glucagon, growth hormone, and cortisol. Without getting into too much detail, just know that they counter the effects of insulin. These five hormones are known as the "stress" hormones. They are secreted in differing amounts during stressful situations and are the reason your blood sugar levels go high when something stressful is happening. Skipping meals, drinking caffeinated beverages, smoking cigarettes, and over-exercising are also stresses to the body and will trigger the stress hormones, too. So, you see that you need to think of more than insulin and food when treating your diabetes.

Here are ten tips for people with type 1 diabetes:

1. It is always more harmful to have low blood sugar reactions than it is to have a high blood sugar level. Do not panic and over-treat with insulin when your blood sugar is high. Take smaller doses of insulin more frequently to bring your blood sugars back down. This is the safest way to avoid going from too high to too low.

2. Treat your blood sugar reaction with any form of sugar such as milk, juice, or icing, but do not try to have low blood sugars so that you can eat sugar! (You can substitute sugars into your meal plan for other carbohydrates.) If you are alert with a low blood sugar, the best choice is to drink whole milk followed by food.

3. You should always expect to go high after a low blood sugar reaction. First, because you have ingested a lot of sugar and second, because the stress hormones are secreted whenever your blood sugar goes very low. Again, do not panic and over-treat your high blood sugar with too much insulin. You will only create another low blood sugar reac-

tion and your blood sugars will yo-yo throughout the day. For the rare times that you do not over-compensate, you will end up with normal blood sugar levels. This is normal, too.

4. Be prepared for low blood sugar reactions. See pages 4–6 of this book for helpful hints. You should always have a glucagon emergency kit on hand. If you do not know what one is, ask your diabetes doctor.

5. Insulin therapy has become smaller multiple injections throughout the day. This is to avoid both high and low blood sugar reactions. After the "honeymoon" period, you will require at least 3 different injection times of insulin.

6. Remember, you can be in ketoacidosis with normal and even low blood sugar levels. If you do not feel well, check your urine ketones frequently.

7. Blood sugar monitors for home use are still one of the biggest breakthroughs in diabetes history. Use your monitor. This will help you avoid low and high blood sugar reactions.

8. Insulin therapy is not just for keeping blood sugar levels normal. Remember that insulin also helps put amino acids and fatty acids into your cells. If you do not take enough insulin or the stress hormones are blocking your insulin action, you can go into ketoacidosis. That is why you must always let your family and your doctor know when you do not feel well enough to eat.

9. Follow sick-day rules when you are ill. See pages 73–77.

10. Exercise decreases your need for insulin. You need to adjust your doses for this.

Having diabetes means that you are missing the hormone insulin. It does not mean anything else. Even though you have to take better care of yourself than your friends without diabetes and take insulin injections, being diabetic is not a handicap. Do not treat yourself that way. Go out and enjoy life like Spike and Bodie Loy do. They have never let having diabetes stop them from doing anything! From motorcycle riding and surfing to vacationing in remote places, these two have done it all. And along with having all this fun, they both have maintained honor grades throughout their academic careers. These two young men are here to tell you that you are just as normal as everyone else. You just have to take a few precautions and realize how full your life can be.

The best of luck to you.

Diana L. Schwarzbein, MD
author of *The Schwarzbein Principle*

Acknowledgments

We thank everyone who contributed time and energy to making this book and especially all our friends who have helped us deal with diabetes all along the way. Thanks to all of our awesome neighbors for learning how to take care of us: the Wildes, the Clems, the MacDonalds, the Sakamotos, the Boccalis, and the whole of Upper Ojai. Thanks to Kevin and Erik and the boys for making sure we eat and paddling us out of the water, and to the guys up at school for the frosting treatment. Thanks to Cheryl for all of her diabetic friendly recipes. Thanks to Dave Brown, Jim Berube, and Jack Smith and all of our teachers and administrators for understanding how a school should handle kids with diabetes. This book would never even have been written if not for the assignment and input from Rick Mohney and Ken Umholtz, so thanks for the homework.

Thanks to Gloria Forgea for all of her help and hope during those first weeks. Thanks to all of the kids and parents from Kids with Diabetes, Inc., for all their priceless input and feedback and their perspectives, especially Patty Conlan for compassion and work with both the book and the group.

Anyone who doesn't have an endocrinologist should start seeing one, and anyone in or around California should start seeing Dr. Diana Schwarzbein. Dr. Diana has been invaluable in helping us understand and live with diabetes, and she helped with the book to boot. Thanks to Dr. Marty Berger and Aunt Gebo for all the editing, input, and especially for putting up with late night calls when we had questions or scares. We want to thank Dr. Chochinov for his help and for working on getting copies of our book into the hands of the kids it was written to help.

Thanks to Grandma Virginia for reviewing the manuscript and for putting up the big bucks so we could continue giving away copies of it. I think we almost have you paid back; the check is in the mail. Thanks to Shed and June Behar for all the editing and help with graphics, to Ellen Shapiro for her input, to David and Jana Hedman for all the color copies and reams of paper we printed our first manuscripts on, and to the whole crew at Mail Boxes Etc., for all of their hard work in pumping out our give-away manuscripts once we hit the "big time."

Thanks also to Timothy Teague for the photos we've adorned our book with at various stages in its never-ending development. Kudos to Larry Hagman on the hill for his friendship, support, and work on editing the book. Thanks to Herman Rush from the other hill for all of his hours editing and all of his support. We owe a lot to Mark Kalmansohn, our lawyer, who donated so much of his time and energy to this project, and to Sherrye Landrum at ADA for treating us well and taking an interest in seeing this project reach fruition. We thank our congressman, Elton Gallegly, for his unswerving support both at home and in Washington. Thanks to Ken Pitzer and Cygnus for hiring me and for their progress with the Glucowatch.

We also thank everyone who worked with us, long before we wrote this book, on research from our ranch. So, thanks to Dr.

Patrick Soon Shiong for getting us involved and excited with islet cell research, to Cobby Oxford the butcher for assisting us with all of the pigs, to Ray Edwards for his work and discovering that Large Whites were the right breed for the job, to Gayle Mortenson from the Pig Improvement Company for her generosity and hard work, to Dave Ochletree for donating his pigs for such a good cause, to John Perry for the use of his stock trailer, and Phil Schmit for using it and tirelessly hauling the 300-pound pigs around the country, to Jake Colborn for building a place to put the porkers, to Gan Nash for completing the whole process with the pigs and Chris for organizing it all, to Margaret Stangeland for always helping, and to Mandy and Wes for their assistance and ambiance. Finally, we want to thank our family for all of their work and input on this book (which at times rivaled ours), especially Mom for her editing, publishing, organizing, and work as our unofficial agent. But far more important, we thank them for their love and devotion for the past 13 years and for always making sure we were all right. We love you.

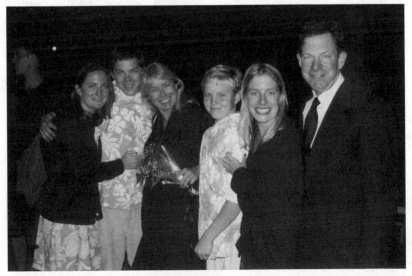

The Loy family at Mom's college graduation

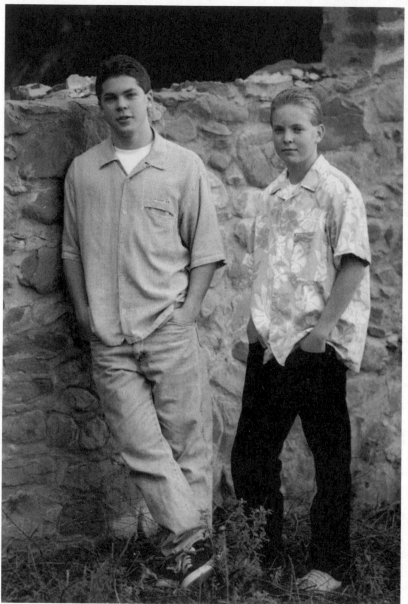

Spike and Bo in front of the Castle

Photo by Timonth Teague

Introduction

Spike Loy was diagnosed at age seven. Bo Loy was diagnosed at age six. Spike and Bo are brothers who have spent the past 15 years living on a 40-acre ranch in rural Upper Ojai, California, with their parents and sisters, Jenny and Mary.

Spike has been managing his diabetes since he was seven years old, and he recently graduated from Stanford University. In his senior year of high school, Spike was valedictorian, homecoming king, ASB Vice President, and a National Merit Scholar. He has been to Ecuador and the Galapagos Islands, Costa Rica, South Africa, and Swaziland among other countries.

He graduated with a degree in human biology and hopes to work in the field of diabetes research. As Spike says, "I am interested in this field because on Thanksgiving day of 1987, I was diagnosed with insulin-dependent diabetes. One year later exactly, on the same day, Thanksgiving day of 1988, my 6-year-old brother Bo was diagnosed as an insulin-dependent diabetic."

Bo graduated from Nordhoff High School in 2000, where he too excelled academically, athletically, and socially. He had a 4.3 grade point average and was the ASB Vice President. He was on the honor roll, served in leadership positions, worked as

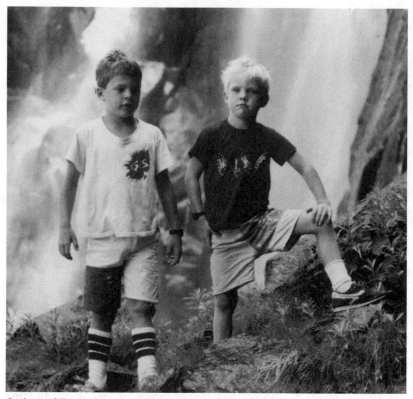
Spike and Bo striking a pose in Yosemite

an associate editor on the school newspaper, and played varsity soccer. He is majoring in biomedical engineering at the University of Southern California. Along with his brother, he has had many adventures around the world, including surfing in Costa Rica and trekking in the South African Veldt. This past summer he spent days backpacking in Yosemite. Bo is an avid surfer and snow boarder. He plays racquetball and enjoys mountain biking in the hills of Upper Ojai.

Bo says, "You can do anything when you have diabetes. Altogether, Spike and I have 29 years of experience dealing with diabetes. We think our experience will help you, and this book will make your life easier. Towards the end of the 1997–98 school year, we began putting down our thoughts about dealing with diabetes. Soon we realized how much we have learned over the years through trial and error. We began sharing this information with other kids. Right away, other diabetics asked for copies, and so our book was born. This book is meant to help kids with diabetes, your families, and your friends. When you have diabetes, you need to develop a support group. This book will show you how. *Getting a Grip on Diabetes* is about what **you can do**!"

YOU CAN DO ANYTHING!

People with diabetes can do everything that anyone else can do. You just have to understand your diabetes and learn about the things you need to do to make your life run smoothly. You will have to be a little more careful about eating and exercising than your friends are. We have put this book together to help

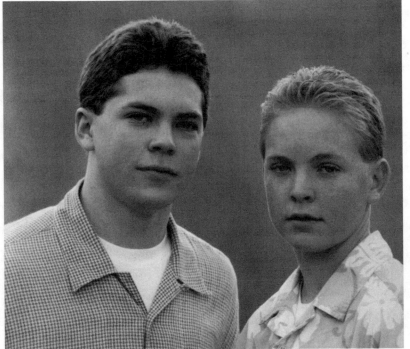

Spike and Bo as newly published authors

Photo by Timonth Teague

you get along more easily in your daily life so you, too, can do everything you want to do.

Inside this book are tips and tricks about how to get along at school, what to do when you're playing sports, what to do when you're feeling a low blood sugar, how to handle traveling around the globe and the extra supplies to take along that will make your trip a breeze, and more.

In the back of the book, you will find documents that we encourage you to reproduce and give to the people you know. We have found that once your friends and their parents, your teachers, and your coaches have an understanding of what diabetes is and the special needs that come along with it, they will be eager to help.

WHAT THE DOC SAYS

Two doctors who work with kids and teens who have diabetes contributed to the "What the Doc Says" sections of this book: Janet Silverstein, MD, of the University of Florida, and Marc Weigensberg, MD, head of pediatric endocrinology at Los Angeles County University of Southern California Medical Center. Dr. Silverstein writes a column for the "Kid's Corner" section of the American Diabetes Association's monthly magazine, *Diabetes Forecast*, and helps run a summer camp for kids with diabetes. Dr. Weigensberg is founder and director of On the Wings of Eagles, a company that promotes a life-issues approach to diabetes in youth and young adults. The program features extended wilderness adventures, family workshops, and ongoing support groups. He currently has a consultative practice in integrative medicine and diabetes care for adolescents and young adults in Beverly Hills, California.

1

What Is Diabetes?

One of your little-known organs is your pancreas. Inside of it are cells called islet cells (pronounced eye-let). Islet cells produce insulin in most people's bodies, but when you have diabetes, they don't. Insulin is like a key that fits into the doors to the cells in your body, unlocks them, and lets sugar (glucose) get into them. If your body doesn't make any insulin keys, all the doors on most of your body's cells stay locked and glucose can't get to where it is supposed to go. When this happens, the sugar builds up in your blood leading to high blood sugar levels, while at the same time, your cells are starving. All the food and drink just passes through your system. This is why you have to pee a lot, and you get dehydrated.

When your pancreas works as it should, every time you eat, it releases just the right amount of insulin. The insulin takes your food to the cells, leaving enough sugar in the blood, so there is back-up. In kids with diabetes, this doesn't work, so we "shoot up" (inject) insulin. Since we put insulin into our body at certain times, it goes to work at certain times, no matter what we eat. If we put a lot of insulin keys into our body but we don't eat any food, the insulin takes all the sugar to our cells at once. There is very little sugar left in our bloodstream, so we get low blood sugar (hypoglycemia). If we don't take any insulin and we eat, our bodies have no insulin keys. The cells can't get the sugar, so it just builds up in our blood, and we get high blood sugar (hyperglycemia).

WHAT THE DOC SAYS:

The type of diabetes that most children and teenagers get is type 1 diabetes because their insulin-producing beta cells in the pancreas have been destroyed by the body's immune system. Usually the immune system fights viruses and bacteria and attacks foreign substances. However, in the case of diabetes, these antibodies attack the beta cells and destroy them. The only way for the body to get the insulin that it needs is by injection with a syringe or by insulin pump. An insulin that you can inhale is likely to be available soon.

Why do we shoot up insulin instead of getting a new pancreas? Because the risk of getting an organ transplant is higher than the benefits. Getting a new organ requires surgery and that can be dangerous. The new islet cell transplants that you hear about in the news are simpler and safer to do, but when you put someone else's body parts into your own, you have to take lots of serious drugs to keep those body parts safe and healthy. The body tries to reject them. Taking daily injections of insulin is actually the easiest and the safest solution to controlling diabetes right now.

How did we become diabetic? One of the leading theories is that for some reason our immune system attacked and destroyed our islet cells. Our white blood cells, which usually attack bacteria and viruses in our bodies, thought that our islet cells looked like viruses and killed them. For this reason we can't just take injections of new islet cells either. Our white blood cells are programmed to think that anything that looks like an islet cell is an enemy, so they attack even new ones.

Currently, scientists are making great strides in conquering diabetes once and for all. Protecting islet cells from white blood cells is one of the most promising approaches and has been used to take human patients off insulin. This is one field of research in which our family has been deeply involved. This research involves transplanting islet cells, protected by little bubble shields, into our bodies. These islet cells work just like the ones we had before diabetes. The bubbles protect the islet cells from white blood cells that would attack. The porous bubbles allow sugar to enter, which stimulates the islets to make insulin. The insulin can then flow out of the bubble into the blood stream while the bubble keeps the white blood cells out and the islets cells alive. We are very hopeful that this research will soon make books like this one obsolete.

HOW DO YOU KNOW WHEN YOU'RE LOW?

If your blood sugar is lower than 80 mg/dl, you might start to feel low. This feeling is caused by low blood sugar; you feel down, and you have less energy. Once it is below 60 mg/dl, you probably will feel it. Most people feel low blood sugars but not everybody does. Whether or not you feel a low blood sugar has to do with the rate of change. If your blood sugar drops rapidly, you're more likely to feel it. If it's dropping gradually, you might miss it. (Since we usually feel it, we are writing from our experience.) As your sugar drops down to around 30 mg/dl, you start feeling quite bad. Sometimes you can mistake high blood sugar feelings for low blood sugar and vice versa.

The best thing to do when you are feeling a little out of it is first to drink or eat something and then test your sugar. If you are really low, the few minutes you spend checking your sugar can be when you pass out, so drinking or eating right away is your best bet. If you are high, well, you will be a little higher after eating, but it's better to be safe than sorry.

When you are low, you may experience:

▪ **Headache**: This is perhaps my first sign of low blood sugar. You may also feel rather lightheaded or a little dizzy. (Headaches are often associated with high sugars as well.)
▪ **Stomachache**: If your stomach feels either knotted up or very empty, chances are that you're low. My stomach usually feels empty when I am around 50–60 mg/dl and gets a severely tight feeling when I am closer to 40 mg/dl.

■ **Shakiness**: If you think you might be low, try holding your hand straight and steady in front of your face. If it is shaking pretty uncontrollably, then you can bet that you are low. The shakier it is, the lower you are. If you don't even feel like you can hold your hand up, then you know you are low and should drink something like fruit juice or milk right away.

■ **Crying, violently upset**: If you get extremely unreasonable and unruly, you may be low. Of course you might just be mad, but if it is first thing in the morning and you get irritable at someone for no good reason, you may be experiencing extremely low blood sugar. However, at this point you probably won't listen to reason, and you may be convinced that you are just plain pissed and won't believe that you are having blood sugar problems. Test your blood and see. After having my mom show me that I was desperately low when I was acting up, I began to believe her. Now I realize that no one is able to make a rational thought when he is low.

There are other signs of more drastic lows, but usually you will not be able to notice them. These include passing out or fainting, not waking up, walking around but not responding, and, at the worst, convulsions. I had never experienced convulsions, but one morning my brother had one. He wouldn't get out of bed—no matter what—so we finally yelled at him and put him on the couch, thinking he was just being stubborn. He didn't touch his breakfast either, and again we blamed it on his stubbornness. Then he laid back down and started twitching. We were able to get him back to normal by squirting frosting under his lip and force-feeding him juice and ice cream. It was hard to get him to eat because when you are "low" you just don't feel like eating anything and definitely don't feel like listening. We didn't send him to school that day either. Hopefully, you can recognize the early warning signs of low blood sugar and avoid major problems altogether by eating a little, so you can get on with your life.

WHAT THE DOC SAYS:

Your blood sugar level is determined by the balance between what you eat, the insulin you take, how much you exercise, and to some degree, your emotional state. Everyone with type 1 diabetes will experience low blood sugar (hypoglycemia) at times. If you take care of it right away by eating or drinking some fast-acting carbohydrate, you can avoid passing out or having convulsions.

Everyone has his or her own unique symptoms of low blood sugar, and you will come to recognize how your own body feels when you're low. Hypoglycemia is somewhat like having your car run out of gas, which then sputters and spits until you fill it again with gas. Your body relies on the fuel of glucose to keep it running, especially your brain, and it will do all it can do to keep glucose flowing to your brain. As your blood sugar drops and you start to run out of fuel, your body secretes glucagon, adrenaline, and other hormones to keep the sugar level up. These lead to the symptoms of shakiness, sweating, and palpitations (heart pounding). If the sugar level continues to drop, you start to experience the symptoms of lack of sugar to the brain, which can include drowsiness, light-headedness, headache, irritability, and hunger. Pay attention to what your symptoms are. Write them down for your teachers and coaches on the sheet (page 104) that tells them what to do to treat your low blood sugar. When you have any symptoms of low blood sugar, it's time to fuel up (eat)! Take 15 g of fast-acting carbohydrate (for example 4 oz. of fruit juice, 6 lifesavers, or 3 glucose tablets) and then test your blood sugar. Expect to feel better in 10–15 minutes. If you don't, eat another 15 g of carbohydrate. Remember to always keep boxed fruit juice, hard candies, glucose tablets, or the tubes of frosting that Bo and Spike use with you at all times for those unpredictable lows.

HOW DO YOU KNOW WHEN YOU'RE HIGH?

High blood sugar is having too much sugar in your blood and your brain. High sugars, 240 mg/dl and above, are not too bad in the short run, but over a long period of time (years), constant high sugars lead to complications. Having too much sugar in your blood makes all of your body's filters work overtime, and they may quit early. Don't be scared by a few high sugars. If you find yourself uncontrollably high for over a week or so, contact your doctor. Remember, if you just can't get your sugars to stabilize perfectly, it is always better to run slightly high than too low.

Here are some things you feel when you're high:

▌ **Thirst**: When your body has too much sugar floating around in it, it needs to balance itself. You get thirsty. It is a good idea to go ahead and drink a lot when this is the case. Water is the best thing, but any sugar-free non-carbonated drink will have a good effect. Drinking a lot leads to some of the other symptoms.

▌ **Need to urinate**: In order to get rid of the sugar, you need to pee frequently. So, if you find yourself having to use the bathroom a couple of times in the same hour, you may want to test your sugar and if it is high, take some insulin. **Safety tip**: Never inject insulin without testing your blood sugar!

- **Your pee is clear**: When there is a lot of sugar in your blood, your urine is very light; there's nothing yellow about it. Check your sugar when you have clear urine. If it stays clear for a long time and your sugar is high, do a urine test and check for ketones (see pages 75–77).
- **Clammy**: I think getting clammy and sweating is just another way your body is trying to regain its balance. My palms often sweat when I have high blood sugar. But they get sweaty sometimes when I get real low, so I always test to be sure which it is.
- **Energy loss**: You might think that with a high blood sugar you would have more energy, but this is not the case. High blood sugar means a lot of sugar is in your blood and your brain but not in your cells where you need it. For this reason you feel pretty lackluster. You need to take insulin, because insulin takes sugar from your blood and delivers it to your cells.

Do growth spurts affect your blood sugar? Often when you are going through growth spurts, your sugars will start to rise. Your normal insulin dose is related to your height and weight. However, when you grow, your body releases hormones that can interfere with insulin action. For this reason, you will often have to increase your dosage by a few units per day. Once the growth spurt is over, though, insulin action will return to normal, and you may experience a few lows because of your increased dosage, but not always. Be ready for this, and carry extra food. Once insulin action returns to normal, bring your dosage slightly back down. You don't have to get an OK from your doctor to change your dosage around just a little. Just make sure the changes make sense and don't put you at risk for hypoglycemia—what we call "crashing." Any large or long-term changes in your insulin dosage should be approved by your doctor, but you don't need to double-check absolutely every time you make a slight change.

WHAT THE DOC SAYS:

High blood sugar (hyperglycemia) can be caused by too much food; not taking enough insulin; or anything that places the body under stress, such as physical illness or a lot of emotional stress. When your blood glucose approaches 200 mg/dl, your kidneys become overloaded and glucose is then lost in the urine, taking water with it. This makes you urinate a lot. This makes you thirsty, so you drink a lot, as your body tries to make up for the extra water lost in the urine. Many people also report feeling tired, or just "different," and knowing their sugar is high. Feeling "clammy" is more commonly a symptom of low blood sugar, but if it is one of your symptoms of high blood sugar, too, please pay attention to it. Although any single high blood sugar is not an emergency, if your high blood sugar won't come down, you may have problems if you also start producing ketones (see pages 75–77), so be careful and take care of it right away. The treatment is generally to take more insulin and drink lots of water or other sugar-free fluids. If you haven't discussed with your doctor exactly how to adjust your insulin doses when your sugar levels are high, it's better to call and ask for advice than to just guess.

2

Getting Organized

THE KIT

The Kit is the name I use for the carrying case in which all of my diabetes products are kept (sometimes I refer to it as "My Life in a Bag"). I carry my kit with me everywhere I go. I take it when I go out to dinner; I take it to school; I take it when I go to spend the night; I take it in the car every time I drive anywhere. Even if I plan on returning home before my next meal, I bring my kit because you never know when you'll be stuck on a freeway or The Big One will hit. (We live in California; I'm thinking earthquake.) It is always best to plan for the worst and to be totally prepared. One of the most important points about the kit is to keep it cool. Ice packs work very well. I keep 3 or 4 in the freezer at all times, so I can replace the pack every day.

Carry your kit with you everywhere you go. The kit contains an insulin kit and a meter kit:

Insulin kit
▌ Insulin bottles
▌ Syringes (plenty extra just in case) or an insulin pen
▌ An injecting device if you use one

Meter kit

- Lancets
- Test strips
- A finger or arm pricker
- A glucose monitor with its test strips (mine is a Freestyle Tracker) and strips that can be read by eye (we use Chemstrips)
- Frosting or glucose tablets (in case you get really low)
- A granola bar (candy bars are often too tempting)
- Identification (something that says who you are and that you have diabetes and also lists emergency contacts and, perhaps, basic procedures on what to do if you are found unconscious) (see page 105)
- Alcohol swabs to sterilize your finger (optional, Bo and I don't use them)

My favorite carrying case is the Medicool's Dia-Pak. I can keep my ice pack separate from the insulin bottles, so I don't have to worry about my insulin getting too cold. I keep my blood testing stuff in a "meter" kit bag. I put my insulin kit in the fridge when I'm home, then both kits go in my carrying case when I go out.

WHAT THE DOC SAYS:

What a great idea to be this organized everyday! The Kit is a diabetes care pack that you can take everywhere, and it contains everything you need to treat low blood sugar, such as fruit juice or 3 glucose tablets. Since these rapid-acting sugar sources last only for a short time, it is important to also have a snack with you that acts slower but lasts longer, such as granola bars or peanut butter or cheese crackers.

Your blood glucose meter and strips are the tools to check your blood sugars. It is helpful to carry a small log book and pen in your kit as well to record your blood sugars. This will help you keep track of patterns of sugar levels. For example, you might be able to see that you have low blood sugar every afternoon after soccer practice. This will help you adjust your insulin dose. Instead of syringes and insulin bottles, many people carry insulin pens with H, R, N, 70/30, or 75/25 insulin in them to make it simpler to take their insulin when they are away from home.

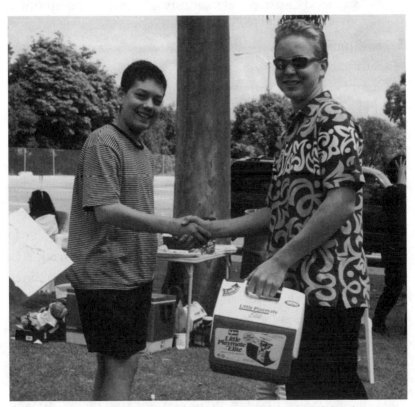

Bo giving a cooler full of the food we keep to a new member of the play group (page 90)

THE COOLER

The Cooler was my single most important possession through-out elementary school and has evolved to adapt to my high school life as well. Personally, I think even kids who don't have diabetes would benefit greatly from always having a well-packed cooler on hand. Fortunately for us, we always have an excuse for keeping one. Every morning I would pack my cooler with my snacks in brown paper bags and my special low-blood-sugar stash and take it to school. There it sat under my desk, and every two hours I would eat one of my snacks. In case I got low, there was always plenty of other stuff in it.

For low blood sugars, my elementary school cooler contained:

- Frosting
- Gatorade
- Granola bars
- Cheez-Its
- Cookies (whatever your favorite kind is)
- Jerky
- Caramels

I thought I was pretty cool when I got into junior high school, and I no longer wanted to take a Little Igloo cooler to school. A lot of the food items can be transferred to a backpack and a locker, but you shouldn't let your cooler go to waste since it has been with you for so long. I carried the same cooler packed with the same goodies and kept it in my favorite teacher's classroom. That way my food was always nearby, and I didn't have to worry about those mean little seventh and eighth graders making fun of my cooler. Once you have a car, you can put a cooler in there, preferably one that plugs into your cigarette lighter, to keep your insulin cool.

My car cooler contains:

- The same foods listed on page 14
- My insulin kit (see pages 11–12)
- Other medication (I am the only one of my friends who always has Benadryl and Tylenol on hand. This has nothing to do with diabetes, but it sure is handy.)

The cooler makes your teachers' lives easier, too. The cooler-in-the-teacher's-class method works best when the cooler also contains a sheet of paper that lists your symptoms of low blood sugar and gives instructions to help you with the situation (see pages 104–105).

WHAT THE DOC SAYS:

Insulin is a protein that breaks down at high temperatures, so you should keep it at a temperature less than 86 degrees but above freezing. Don't leave insulin in your car in the heat of the summer. If you do leave your insulin someplace where it has gotten very hot, throw away that bottle and get a new one from the pharmacy.

Bo and Spike keep frosting and Gatorade in their cooler to treat low blood sugars quickly. Once they are feeling a bit better, they eat the Cheez-Its, cookies, or jerky to keep their blood sugar up over a longer period of time. Jerky is primarily protein and fat and will be absorbed slowly. That's why it is not the food to use first to treat low blood sugar.

THE DIABETES DRAWER

Just as the cooler and the kit are convenient places to keep all of our diabetic necessities when we are away from home, certain kitchen drawers are ideal places for storing things at home. Our Diabetes Drawer is right under the counter top where we draw our insulin and shoot up.

The Diabetes Drawer contains:

- Needles
- Lancets
- Alcohol swabs
- Finger or arm pricker
- Injector
- Blood glucose meter kit (meter, strips, lancets, and pricker)
- Our kits (when not in use, minus the ice pack and the insulin, which go in the refrigerator). Do not put your meter in the fridge!

Insulin needs to be kept cool at all times. When insulin gets too hot, it goes bad. If you are experiencing high sugars, it may be because your insulin is bad due to overheating. Throw it out, and start a new bottle. Sometimes when you start a new bottle, you may experience lows because the insulin is more potent than the insulin in the old bottle.

WHAT THE DOC SAYS:

Organization is important for everyone, but especially if you have diabetes. Once you get organized as Bo and Spike suggest, you have more time to do other things you want to do without wasting time trying to find the supplies that you need when a situation arises or it's time to go to school.

It is true that new insulin is sometimes more potent than old insulin. But if you don't mix your insulin well enough, the active insulin molecules may settle in the bottle and make

---

the end of the vial more potent. Studies show that you need to roll the vial about 45 times to mix the insulin.

How Can You Use the Refrigerator-Freezer?

▮ **Use the butter drawer in your refrigerator for your insulin.** The butter drawer is ideal because it closes. When we forget to close it, our insulin often flies out when we open the door and once in awhile breaks. Using the butter drawer properly can save money (and the mockery family members enjoy bestowing on you). Use a specific shelf in the freezer door for ice packs. This way you will always know where they are. Every time you come home, unpack your kit and return all insulin to the butter drawer and ice packs to the freezer door shelf. This will ensure that you always have frozen ice packs and potent insulin. Put your meter kit back in the Diabetes Drawer.

▮ **Keep a glucagon kit in your fridge.** Glucagon is like a security blanket. If you are ever drastically low, someone can inject you with glucagon to raise your blood sugar. See page 120 for more about glucagon.

▮ **When you're at other people's homes, go ahead and put your insulin kit in their refrigerator.** This will keep everything cool, and you won't lose anything. If you can remember to retrieve it, put the ice pack in their freezer, but keeping it with the kit in the fridge will serve your purpose as well. Keep your meter kit in your backpack or cooler.

Having everything organized and standardized makes my life much easier and eliminates the chance of forgetting to shoot up. You would think that might be hard to forget to do, but once you break your routine (like when summer starts or when you're at a friend's house), you do things in the wrong order. The more systematic your insulin setup is, the less chance there is for error.

WHAT THE DOC SAYS:

Glucagon is a hormone that works as the opposite to insulin by raising blood sugar. Everyone with diabetes needs an up-to-date glucagon kit in the refrigerator to be used by a family member or housemate in case you have a severely low blood sugar and you are unable to take sugar by mouth on your own. Check your refrigerator now—if you don't have glucagon or your kit has expired, call your doctor's office for a new prescription. Everyone in the house needs to know when and how to use glucagon.

3

Elementary School

I was diagnosed with type 1 diabetes when I was seven years old, just a month after I started the second grade. I made it through elementary school with hardly any diabetes-related problems. The main reason was because my family let every single person at the school (and in the entire town for that matter) know that I had diabetes and informed them what to do if I were to experience low blood sugars.

Here are a few things you and your parents should do:

- **Arrange parent-teacher conferences**. Before school starts, meet with all of the teachers and faculty at the school and instruct them not only on worse-case-scenario procedures but also on the daily needs of a kid with diabetes, such as needing to eat in class and using the restroom frequently when blood sugars are high.
- **Tell all of your friends**. Whenever someone comes over to your house or every time your parents pick you up at school, have them tell your friends a few things. They should know that if you were ever to "fall asleep" or lose consciousness, they should squirt a little frosting on your gums and get an

adult. They should also know why they must never eat your special food.

■ **Have special food at the school.** I always had granola bars and caramels in my desk just in case. I also had my little Igloo Cooler under my teacher's desk filled with all sorts of food so I could recover from a low. I had food like apple juice, snack crackers, more granola bars and caramels, beef jerky, and any other of my favorite foods—no one wants to eat something gross when they have a low blood sugar.

■ **Take your cooler on the bus and on all field trips.**

■ **Have a granola bar in your pocket during assemblies.**

One of these points that I cannot stress enough is to let all of your friends know that you are a diabetic. **Tell them what to do when you need sugar.**

One day out on the playground, I just sat down and felt really dizzy. My good friend Kevin knew there was something wrong with me. He started talking to me and walked me to the office, called my mom, and started to feed me my caramels. Sometimes no grown-ups are around, and you might feel too bad to go all the way to your cooler or desk, but your friends can always help you.

We gave every teacher and the principal a copy of my **symptoms** (page 104) and a clear plastic baggie filled with: a small Cake Mate frosting, a 6 oz. can of apple juice, a granola bar, and peanuts. It helped the teachers know what to do if we got low in class.

WHAT THE DOC SAYS:

The take-home lesson here is clear: Don't isolate yourself. I've known teens with diabetes who felt embarrassed,

---

ashamed, or just different from everyone else, and there-fore, they didn't want to tell others about their condition. While these feelings are understandable, isolating yourself or trying to hide your diabetes is really not in your best interest. First of all, virtually everyone has something that he or she feels this way about, whether it's a physical trait, a personality feature, or just a weird family member. Be proud of who you are and what makes you unique, even your dia-betes. When you tell others, you give them a chance to know you better, let them be available if you truly need help (such as if you get low), and may even have a profound effect on them that you could never foresee.

For example, my best friend in junior high school had dia-betes, and I truly believe that knowing him and seeing what he had to do to care for himself on a daily basis gave me a deep respect for him and his family. He was one important reason that I eventually became a pediatric endocrinologist. Thank you, Steve.

–MW

4

Outdoor School

All through elementary school, the one thing I looked forward to more than anything else was attending Outdoor School. (It's like going to camp with your school. You sleep in a tent or cabin, and you're kind of roughing it.) When it came time to go, though, I thought that I might not be able to make it. I was completely wrong. I was fortunate enough to have my mother come along as a chaperone. If your parents have the time and money, I strongly suggest they go on all of these excursions or at least spend a day training a teacher or other parent who will be going. I was extremely grateful that my mother came. Diabetes places a lot of responsibility on all of us kids and any time that we can be a little freer is extremely valuable.

There were a lot of things to do before heading off to Catalina. You can use what we did to plan your own camping or outdoor school experience.

■ **Contact the camp beforehand.** Let the supervisors and counselors at any camp you are going to attend know that you are diabetic and give them clear instructions on what to do if you have low blood sugars.

- **Look into eating arrangements.** Be sure that there will always be food available and that the people in charge know to give you access whenever necessary.
- **Bring along plenty of extra insulin.** Murphy's Law applies especially well to diabetes. Whenever you mix insulin and backpacks and rocky hikes, chances are something will break. Be sure to bring plenty of extra insulin, syringes, injection devices, or whatever you use, and remember to let the camp know you will need to refrigerate your insulin before you get there. Advance notice always helps.
- **Bring extra food.** Always take your own special snack food; nobody understands what special food you need better than

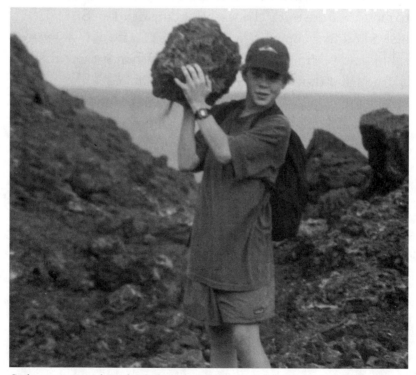

Spike, acting tough in the Galapagos Islands

you. Wherever you go, you need extra food, even if it is at a camp where they tell you to keep food out of tents because of bears or other scavengers. The counselors will be able to tell you what kind of food and packaging is required to prevent or contain the smells that attract animals. This is another reason for contacting them before you go to camp.

■ **Be especially careful of cold water**. At Catalina we went for a night snorkel. Despite wearing full wetsuits—beaver tails and all—I still became excessively cold, and my sugars dropped significantly. It's OK to swim in to shore early. Just tell an adult that you need to go in for food because of your diabetes and be sure to swim in with a friend.

The key thing to do when going to a camp or outdoor school or anything of that nature is to let the people running it know about your special needs well ahead of time. This will help prepare them, and they will help you gain access to anything that you may need while you're there. At Catalina I had to get food out of the cafeteria during "closed time" on several occasions. Everything was fine, though, because everybody knew that I had permission.

For five days camping on Catalina, I took a small suitcase filled with 1 box each of Wheat Thins, Cheez-Its, and chocolate chip cookies, 3 bottles of Gatorade, 12 granola bars, 5 bags of beef jerky, 1 tub of frosting, 3 tubes of frosting (for my wetsuit), 1 small jar of peanut butter, a jar of peanuts, plastic baggies, paper bags, and a marking pen. Each morning we prepared snacks for 10 AM, 2 PM, 4 PM; and 8 PM; put them in bags; wrote the snack time on the bag; put them into my backpack; and I was off.

WHAT THE DOC SAYS:

I highly recommend an experience in the outdoors, whether at an organized diabetes summer camp or through some other program. For the last several years, I have had the privilege of leading teenagers with diabetes into the wilderness on backpacking and whitewater canoeing adventures. Not only can you do these things safely with diabetes, but you may find "getting away from it all" a good opportunity to learn how flexible you can really be with your diabetes. The challenges of a different environment offer a great way to learn more about yourself and your diabetes self-care. The best advice about such experiences is to plan ahead. By considering all of your needs and discussing them ahead of time with the camp or program staff, you can set up a situation where you can have a terrific experience in the great outdoors.

5

Sports

When I first found out that I had something called diabetes, I was afraid that my short-lived sports career had, perhaps, come to an early end. I couldn't have been any further from the truth. With only very minor alterations to my schedule, I was able to continue playing soccer, baseball, and basketball, so diabetes didn't affect my abilities one bit. I was still able to make the all-star teams for soccer and baseball (I was never any good at basketball to begin with).

TEAM SPORTS

Here are some of the things that kids with diabetes have to do a little differently when playing team sports:

▌ **Just like at school, tell everyone involved: coaches, players, other parents, even referees**. Diabetes is certainly nothing to be ashamed of—it can't keep you from anything—and definitely not something to keep a secret.

▌ **Check your blood sugar before each practice and each game**. If you have low blood sugar, DO NOT start playing.

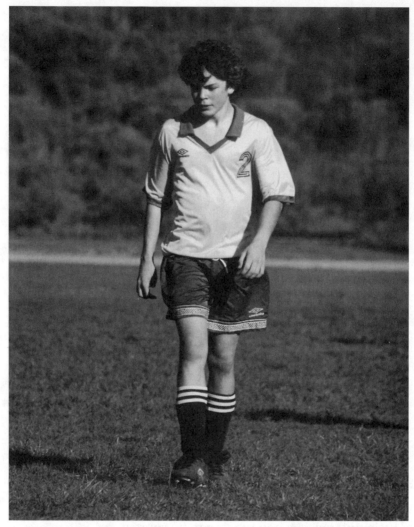

Spike, tired after a soccer match

Exercise lowers your sugar fairly rapidly, so you need to eat and start feeling better before you start to play. (It should only take 5 or 10 minutes to get your sugar up.) You also shouldn't go out on the field if your sugar is very high (above 300 mg/dl). It seems logical to get exercise to help bring your sugars down, but very high blood sugars and exercise just make you feel bad. Take a little insulin, one or two units (very little—it's better to be high than low), and eat a little. **Always eat something when you take insulin, even when you are high.** Test again in 15 minutes to see if you've lowered your blood sugar enough to play.

▮ **During breaks in the game, quarters, innings, and half time, eat a little something.** I always drink Gatorade at quarters and maybe eat a little granola bar at halftime. You don't have to come out of a game to eat, just run to the sideline. Tell the referee what you are doing and there won't be any problems.

▮ **Sometimes you need to eat some real food.** If you are playing just after a big meal and just took a lot of insulin or if you are getting lots of exercise, you may need to eat a meal between or even during your game. I always liked McDonald's Chicken McNuggets because you can eat them one at a time. Your friends might beg you for some (especially if it's been a long tournament), but just tell them that you have to eat it, and they will understand.

The three best ways of controlling diabetes are with insulin, diet, and exercise. Your blood sugar may be a little bit wacky when you start playing a sport after a month or more off, but soon your athletics will help bring your sugars down to a totally normal level. By just being a little bit more careful and by eating a little bit more than you used to, you can play as many sports as you like and may be an all-star in every one of them!

WHAT THE DOC SAYS:

Spike and Bo are right on. Diabetes will not keep you from participating in sports or other activities. To get the most

continued

---

from your sports activities, you'll need to check your blood sugar before and after you exercise to see the effect of exercise on your blood sugar. If you have ½–1 hour before an athletic event, you could eat a granola bar for the carbohydrates. If it is 2 hours before the game, you could have a low-fat, moderate-protein, high-carbohydrate meal, such as cereal, banana, and milk for breakfast or pizza and salad for lunch or dinner. A turkey or chicken sandwich would work well, too. The carbohydrates in these meals will be working just about the time you are playing.

If you are going to play strenuously for an hour or less, a box of juice (8 oz.) or Gatorade should keep your blood sugar up. A good rule of thumb is: carbohydrates raise your blood sugar for the first 1–2 hours, protein for the next 2–4 hours, and fat for the 4–6 hours after the food is eaten. McDonald's McNuggets, like most fast foods, are very high in fat, so try to eat an amount that fits into your meal plan.

Remember that exercise makes your body more sensitive to insulin, so you may get low blood sugars immediately after exercise and also later on, when your insulin action is peaking. So, it is wise to take an extra bedtime snack or snack bar with cornstarch on the days that you get lots of exercise.

Check your blood sugar before the game. If it is 100 mg/dl or less, have 15 g of carbohydrate right away and again every hour. If it is 170 mg/dl, have 15 g of carbohydrate in an hour and again every hour. If it is 200 mg/dl, go ahead and play, but check your blood sugar every hour. If it is 240 mg/dl, check your urine for ketones, and if there are none present, then go ahead and play, checking your blood sugar every hour.

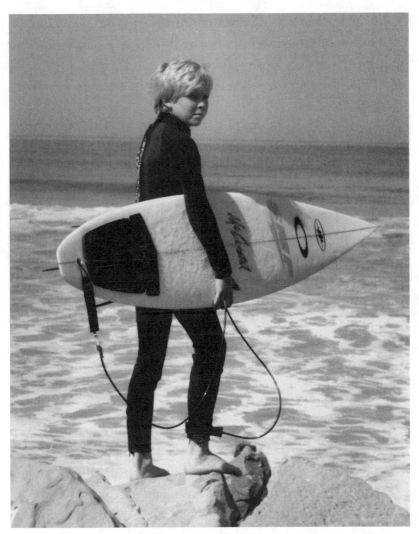

Bo, ready to surf at Pitas Point

SURFING

Bo and I have surfed since we were six years old. It is my favorite sport and also the one where I have run into the most complications due to diabetes. The generally cold waters of Ventura County are especially draining on my body, and I have found that even with a wetsuit, it is not wise to stay out in the line-up for much more than an hour before having a little snack. Your body burns a lot of calories when you're paddling your heart out (feels like for your life—sometimes it is) in ocean water that's barely 50 degrees.

Here are some things I do now to avoid the lows:

- **Stock up on fast food every single time I go to the beach**. Always eat a burger or a taco before paddling out and each time you paddle back in. It takes a lot of energy for anyone to surf all day.
- **Roll up a tube of frosting in the sleeve of your wetsuit**. If you ever have a severe low while in the water, a tube of frosting can be what it takes to get you back in to shore.
- **Take a cooler**. Filling a cooler full of food and bringing it to the beach can save you a lot of money at McDonalds and Taco Bell. I still recommend buying and eating some protein-filled food before you paddle out, though. Keep a glucagon kit in your cooler.
- **Never stay out in the line-up for more than an hour**. Even if it's the best surf you have ever seen, you need to go in and **eat frequently**. This will ensure that you are feeling great and can surf your best on the best days.
- **If you feel low, tell someone you are surfing with**. If you have diabetes, **never surf alone**. There is too much potential for getting into trouble. If you ever feel low when you're out in the water, just tell your friend or even a complete stranger if he or she is the only one around and can help you get in.

I have never actually passed out in the surf, but I have had some scary moments. After a rather large wipe-out and at least ten seconds under the surface, I paddled back out past the breakers. I was pretty cold and figured that was why I was shaking so much. Then my leg began to cramp up something fierce, but I rubbed it, and about 3 minutes later, I had control of it again. I was shaking pretty good by now and could hardly hold my head off the board. I had enough sense to turn toward shore and start paddling, so the white-water washed me in. I left my board on the beach, climbed the stairs to my friend's beach house, and started eating ice cream. I didn't feel normal for more than an hour and a full meal or two later. I thought I was just cold, but my mom told me that after I had come in, she had tested my blood sugar, and it was a scant 20 mg/dl. I was pretty lucky, but I wish that I had had enough sense to just tell somebody out in the line-up.

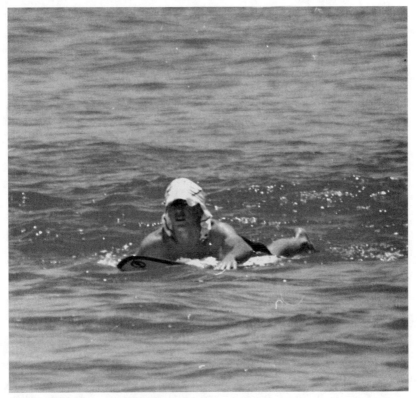

Spike, paddling in, Baja, Mexico

I learned a lesson that day: if you are feeling odd or bad or different, tell somebody.

WHAT THE DOC SAYS:

Life offers you many exciting, fun, and adventuresome experiences. You can do them all with diabetes, but please take the time to think ahead, and don't dismiss the risks of certain activities just because you don't want to be different. The advice in this section shows a nice balance between adventure and reasonable precautions, and you can apply it to other adventurous activities. Plan ahead, and don't be afraid or embarrassed to ask for help if you need it. Sometimes we think we have to do things on our own or else somehow we've failed. In fact, we all depend on each other in some way or other, so if you get into a difficult situation in the surf, or on a mountain, or wherever you find yourself, just ask for help.

MOTORCYCLE AND BICYCLE RIDING

Motorcycle riding is a unique sport. There is more than just physical exertion involved. It takes a lot of mental and physical work to ride for long periods of times. It can be really cold or really hot out, and because you can travel so far on a bike, you must be prepared.

Spike and I follow this routine for both motorcycle and bicycle riding.

■ **Pack food.** The most important thing to remember is to take enough food when you go for a ride. For instance, if you are going out for a 2-hour ride, 1 hour down the trail and 1 hour

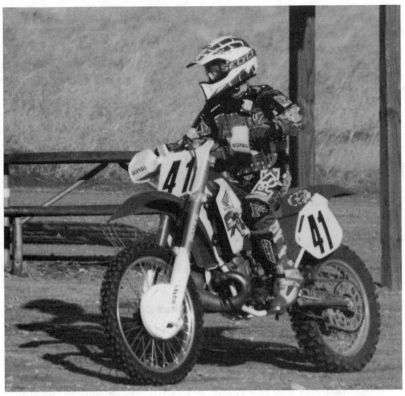

Bo, riding in the desert

back, you have to be prepared to be able to walk back. It may be miles. Plan for the worst. Take enough food with you in your butt pack, so that if your bike breaks down or if you have a wreck, you can get back to civilization. Take a glucagon kit. I always carry a large butt pack.

▌ **Check your sugar before you start riding**. You may also want to reduce your insulin when you're riding.

▌ **Calorie up before riding**. I find that I can eat twice as much as usual when I'm riding all day, because the sport uses so much energy.

▌ **Try a camelback**. For any long rides, you'll appreciate a camelback to carry liquids. It's a small backpack that holds liquids with a long straw to your mouth so you can drink while you're riding.

- **Never ride alone.** If your bike won't make it back, you can always hop on your buddy's bike and get a ride back. My friends always carry a tube of frosting with them just in case I get low, and I'm not in shape to help myself. The frosting perks you up enough to eat a real snack.
- **Prepare for accidents and injury.** If you should have an accident that requires a ride to the hospital, you'll have your kit and snack food right with you in your butt pack.
- **Know what to do at the hospital.** If you should have to go to the hospital, take your kit filled with your insulin and your meter kit with your blood testing stuff. Things will go much more smoothly if you and your parents monitor your blood sugar while the doctor takes care of stitches or broken bones. Injuries can cause your sugar to soar or crash— usually crash.

It was January 17, 1994, the day of the big Northridge quake, here in Southern California. After the excitement of the earthquake, I went for a trail ride. I was taking it easy on my bike, just going up a hill in some soft dirt when I simply laid the bike over. The chain caught my leg cutting through my jeans from knee to ankle. It splayed my shin open, a 6-inch gash to the bone. I was able to ride home to get help.

On the way to the hospital, I had my butt pack with my kit and snacks. We were able to test my blood sugar in the car. It dropped a little, and I needed some of that snack. In the emergency room, while the doctor irrigated my wound and got ready to sew it up, my mom used my kit to keep testing my blood to monitor my blood sugar. She gave me food and Gatorade when I needed it. We probably did 3 blood tests during the emergency room visit. My sugar kept dropping, and I kept eating and drinking.

BACKPACKING

Backpacking is a lot of fun, but there are a few extra things you need to take with you and a few things you need to know. You need to take enough food, so if you get lost or end up spending more time away from civilization than you planned, you have enough food to make it. I always carry extra food for an additional 24 hours. Remember, when you are out in the woods away from people, stores, and medical care, you will need to take extra precautions. **Do not hike alone.** Tell someone where you will be, protect your kit so nothing gets broken banging around in your backpack, and carry extra insulin. Don't exhaust yourself, do eat frequently, and filter the water. You don't need to get sick.

Besides warm clothes and water, here's what I pack:

▪ **Granola bars.** Put them in both your backpack and your pockets where they are easy to reach.

- **Gatorade**. This is a good drink for low blood sugars. It is also a good way to keep your body hydrated while hiking or backpacking. You can carry Gatorade in a powder form, then all you have to do is add water. It's lighter to carry the powder.
- **Beef jerky and peanuts**. Jerky is lightweight and a good source of protein. Jerky and peanuts are good long-acting foods to have when you'll be using up lots of energy.
- **Trail mix**. Make sure you don't abuse trail mix. Trail mix often has a lot of chocolate, raisins, and other dried fruit mixed in. These can be good for low blood sugars but shouldn't be eaten freely. Be aware of what is in your trail mix, and stay away from the ones that are packed with sweets.
- **Kit**. Keep your kit out of the sun. Keep it cool if the weather is hot, or warm if you're hiking in the snow. If you're camping in the snow, sleep with it in your sleeping bag.
- **Glucagon**. Carry your glucagon kit. Tell your friends to inject you with glucagon if you should pass out and the frosting doesn't work. Make sure they know exactly where it is or let them carry it. There is no 911 out in the wilderness.

Although I highly recommend getting plenty of exercise, backpacking requires some preparation. You use extreme amounts of energy, especially when you're at high altitudes, carrying a heavy pack, or when it's cold. Before you go backpacking, think about these things:

- **Calories**. You'll need up to twice as many calories when backpacking.
- **Never hike alone**. Hike with a friend. Friends can help carry the extra food you'll need.
- **Reduce your insulin**. Start out using less insulin. If it's a serious trip, you will use less insulin. I usually inject only half of

my regular short-acting dose before a day of backpacking. Check your blood sugar often. This way you'll know what you need to eat and how much insulin you should inject.

■ **Snacks.** Pack snacks in separate bags and write the time to eat the snack on each bag. When you change your routine, sometimes you forget to eat. This will help you remember.

Note: Warm muscles use up sugar independent of insulin. After a day of heavy exercise, your muscles will continue to use sugar for hours. You will need to use far less short-acting insulin at dinner. Be prepared to wake up and check a midnight blood sugar level, and watch for lower blood sugar levels for the 24 hours after you return home.

WHAT THE DOC SAYS:

Backpacking into the wilderness can be a life-changing experience that will challenge you to be your best and give you many rewards. But it does add many variables to your usual diabetes self-care plan with which you may not be familiar. I would offer the following practical tips based on my personal experiences in the backcountry with teens with diabetes.

1. With the increased activity, temperature extremes, and high altitude often found in the backcountry, hypoglycemia is quite common. Be prepared to check your sugar frequently, including late at night, or maybe even in the middle of the night, especially if you've spent a long day hiking. Carry **plenty** of "low food" to treat hypoglycemia. This could be raisins, dried fruit, nutrition

continued

bars, or glucose tablets. Keep your gear well organized, and always know where the low foods are.

2. Be very knowledgeable about your diabetes, or go with someone who is knowledgeable. Such variables as extreme exercise, altitude, or climate mean you may need to significantly change your usual insulin dose rapidly. Having to reduce your insulin dose by 20–50% is not unusual.

3. If you go to high altitudes too quickly, you may experience symptoms of altitude sickness, which can mimic low blood sugar. Drink plenty of water to prevent dehydration. Drink even before you are thirsty.

4. Since you may be far from conventional medical care, know basic first aid, or travel with someone who does.

5. Some glucose meters don't work as well at high altitudes. Check with the manufacturer before you leave home.

6. Never, ever hike alone. A low blood sugar on the trail should not turn a wonderful experience in nature into a disaster.

7. Always carry some form of identification stating that you have diabetes and an instructional sheet on what to do if you can't help yourself.

MORE ABOUT HEAVY EXERCISE

(We are talking about hard, prolonged exercise here.)

The Most Important Thing We Can Share with You

Lower your dinnertime insulin dose after you've done extreme exercise. You will also want to adjust your insulin dose down before heavy exercise.

Heavy exercise is a day of sports tournaments, snow boarding or skiing all day, racquetball, surfing for 3 hours or more, motorcycle riding all day, or bike riding half a day. It also applies to an afternoon of high school practice for active sports like football, basketball, swim team, soccer, or track. (This doesn't apply to a game of pick-up basketball in the driveway.)

When you have diabetes and you exercise all day, you will need to stop and think about just how much short-acting insulin you should take at dinner. Each sport you play will have slightly different calorie and insulin requirements.

▪ **Exhaustion calls for a different routine**. This is because all day your muscles have been using up the sugar from your meals. The sugar that was stored in your muscle tissue has been used up, too. For the next 8 hours or so, in the middle of the night, while you are sleeping, your muscles will be taking sugar out of your blood stream and putting it back into storage. Low blood sugar can result.

▪ **After exercising all day, you need to avoid getting drastically low in the middle of the night**. Eat dinner, cut down your insulin dose by 1/2 or more, and eat a good snack with protein and carbs before going to sleep. (Eat a snack before bed even if your sugar is a little high, because your warm muscles will use it up during the night.)

▪ **Think about a soccer game**. Soccer is a running game. You might run 3 or 4 miles during a soccer game. If it's a morning game and I usually take 8 units of short-acting insulin, I'll take only 4 units. After the game, at lunchtime I'll test. If I usually take 5 units of short-acting insulin at lunch, I'll only take 2. By dinnertime, after a morning game, I'll test and take my normal dose.

▪ **Now consider a soccer tournament**. You might have three soccer games on the same day with more games to come on the next day. You might run 8 or 10 miles on a tournament day. Before the first game, I cut my insulin dose in half. I snack at quarters, and at halftime. I have a huge lunch and test. If my sugar is low, I skip my noontime insulin. I continue snacking and eating for energy throughout game two and game three. By dinnertime my sugar might be climbing. Let's say it's around 180 mg/dl. **But after heavy exercise your dinnertime insulin dose will be different. It will be lower.** I will cut down my short-acting insulin dose to half or less.

WHAT THE DOC SAYS:

Exercise lowers blood sugar independently of insulin. This effect can be so great with extreme exercise that some diabetic professional athletes will take only extremely small insulin doses before a big game. The actual effect of heavy exercise on blood sugar can differ greatly from person to person and the increase in glucose use following exercise can last for several days. Whatever changes you make in your insulin dose to compensate for exercise, be sure to test your sugar afterward to learn about how your body responds when you push it. If you have any questions, be sure to ask your diabetes health care professional.

6

Pursuing Academics

Diabetes doesn't have to affect your academic schoolwork as long as you keep even moderate control of it. I was able to become the valedictorian of my high school and get a 1550 on my SAT. Diabetes in no way challenged my academics. A few precautions can be taken, however, to assure that it doesn't hamper you in your schooling.

Some things to do to keep your scores up:

▌ **Always bring extra food and snacks when taking major tests (finals, SAT, AP).** I typically bring a granola bar or two and a bottle of Gatorade to snack on while testing and a whole snack (crackers, string cheese, banana) to eat during the breaks in the tests.

▌ **Inform the test proctor of your needs.** Some of the tests have specific instructions against eating. If you tell the administrator that you have diabetes and don't make a big deal out of eating, there won't be a problem. If there is a problem, you don't have to take the test, and you can notify the test administrators. You do have to be treated a little differently some times.

- **Remember to eat**. Even if you don't feel low, you should "graze." You may think it strange, but strenuous brain activity actually has the same effect on my sugar as physical activities. My sugars drop significantly when I compete or test without eating. Don't worry if other students are not allowed to eat in test situations, you **basically have to**.

- **If you feel low during a test, inform your teacher or the test administrator.** In the classroom, your teacher will have already been informed of your condition and its complications, so you will probably be able to retake the test. At standardized national tests, you may have to contact the testing center for information regarding their policy, but you are entitled to a retake.

- **Let your teacher know.** If you were having low sugars or working on getting rid of ketones and it kept you from doing your homework, let your teacher know the next day. Never use diabetes as an excuse if it didn't really affect anything, but if it did, don't be afraid to tell your teacher. They know that your health is more important than one assignment and will undoubtedly let you make it up.

If you feel bad, always remember to take care of your health before anything else, even final exams. If you can't make up a test, remember that a grade is just a mark on a piece of paper. Five years down the road it won't mean a thing, but the way you feel will. I can count on one hand the times that I have had to stop doing something academic because of my blood sugar. Diabetes may give you tiny setbacks, but it can't keep you from any kind of scholarly achievement whatsoever.

WHAT THE DOC SAYS:

This section raises interesting issues regarding diabetes and special treatment. While diabetes may not be a disability in the classic use of the word, the reality is that there may be certain circumstances where special treatment is a medical necessity. My best advice is to be realistic about your situation and ask only for what you truly need. Don't use your diabetes to manipulate situations falsely in your favor. The balanced approach suggested in this section will serve you well.

7

Eating Out

Going out to dinner really isn't much different at all when you have diabetes. As in most other activities though, you'll need to be a little more responsible. You can still eat most everything on the menu—just stay away from too much food with lots of sugar and match your carbohydrates with protein (see page 95). When you go out to dinner, you might as well treat yourself to something you enjoy like French fries.

What to do when you go out to dinner:

■ **Never shoot up too early**. You want to make sure food will be available when you need it. At restaurants you never know how long it will take before you are served. To avoid lows I take my insulin after the food arrives. Ideally you should shoot up about 15–30 minutes before you eat (depending on what type of short-acting insulin you take), but at restaurants that's impossible to gauge. Sometimes, if I have high blood sugar, I inject my insulin a few minutes after ordering my food but even that is taking a chance. What if they lose my order?

- **Don't be afraid to tell your waitress that you absolutely must have some food.** If you shot up too early or are just having a low for other reasons, tell the waitress that you are diabetic and need food right away. Maybe you can tip her a little extra (don't worry about that until after your sugar has come back up).

- **Always bring a little bit of your own food.** When you are going out to eat, you still carry your trusty granola bar in your pocket. This will keep you from having to demand food and allow you to shoot up earlier. If your food is long in coming, you will have some backup right there.

- **Don't be shy about shooting up.** I have known some diabetics who hide their injections out of some notion of politeness. Don't be afraid to shoot up at the table. You can do it without attracting a lot of attention. Or you may want to ask if anyone is squeamish and tell them what you are doing. Most people are extremely interested and even mesmerized by it. I try to get my friends to do it for me. I draw the insulin; then they can inject in my arms and give my legs and hips a break.

- **Watch your sugar.** Restaurants load any sweet food with tons of extra sugar. Desserts are a luxury not a necessity, so I avoid them most of the time and maybe have a bite of my date's or my friend's. On very special occasions, I sometimes treat myself, but I don't usually eat a whole dessert. After avoiding sugar for so long, I noticed that really sweet things lose their appeal—kind of a plus when you have diabetes or just want to be healthy.

Just remember to go ahead and tell people that you are a diabetic. Shoot up only when you know food is coming, and then eating out won't be any different than it is for nondiabetics.

WHAT THE DOC SAYS:

The best lesson here is, again, don't be shy about who you are and what you need to do to care for yourself. Next, even if you are very knowledgeable about nutrition and are great at counting carbs (see page 99), it can be pretty tricky to estimate the carbohydrate content or portion sizes of restaurant food. Do your best, but be prepared to supplement with extra insulin if you undershoot the insulin dose.

8

Traveling the Globe

The time to be most careful is when you are far away from home and far away from people who know you have diabetes and know what to do. You must be more careful, but you can still have the time of your life traveling around the country and the world. As long as you take a few medical precautions and pack a little bit extra, you can avoid any real problems.

Plan ahead to be safe when traveling. Here's what we do:

■ **Pack lots of extra insulin and other diabetic supplies**. What I usually do is pack my normal kit (page 11) and then pack one or two more duplicate kits (depending on the duration of my trip and how far I am going). You shouldn't put all of your extra insulin in the same place though, because if one bottle is lost, stolen, or broken, then all of them will be too.

■ **Always carry your insulin on you when you fly somewhere**. The luggage compartments on many flights either get extremely cold or hot or both, and this is not a good thing for insulin, especially when you are going to be out of the country for a week or two.

- **Let the management at all hotels know that you need to use a freezer for ice packs.** I always freeze extra ice packs and keep one with my insulin. I hesitate to put my insulin in refrigerators in a hotel kitchen because of the chance that it may be lost, broken, or stolen. You can always buy more ice packs though. Also, try to get a room with a mini bar refrigerator. They work perfectly for insulin.
- **Let the flight attendant on any flight know that you are a diabetic.** This way you will be assured food when you need it, and it is always nice to have some extra peanuts. You can request a special meal several days before you fly, but ask what it will be in case you don't like the food choices.
- **Pharmacies have to give you insulin and needles.** If a pharmacy has what you need in stock, you don't need a prescription to get it. If you are totally without your insulin, syringes, or blood sugar testing equipment, tell the pharmacist that it is an emergency, and he or she will help you out. Show identification that you have diabetes and, if necessary, be stubborn until you get what you need. It's a good idea to have a letter from your doctor or a prescription form stating that you have diabetes and what you need. Be aware that insulin in other countries is not the same potency as ours. You'll have to adjust and inject a different amount to the get the effect you need if you use the syringes that you bring with you. Syringes are different sizes in other countries, too. If you use syringes that you buy in the same place you buy the insulin, you can take the same amount of the insulin that you usually do. Ask your doctor for help with this.
- **Take lots of food with you wherever you go.** When I go on big trips, I take an extra suitcase just for food. I take enough beef jerky, Gatorade, crackers, and granola bars to live off for the entire trip if need be. It's a bit of a hassle, but I think I

would probably do it now even if I weren't diabetic. (I like to eat.)

■ **Carry a glucagon kit**. Also carry directions for how to use it.
■ **Wear a medical ID and carry a diabetes ID card**.

It is especially important to always have food on you. On our flight home from South Africa, the flight attendants' union was on strike. The in-flight meal consisted of a bag of peanuts and water for a 15-hour flight. That could have been a very bad thing, but Bo and I had plenty of food in our backpacks, so there was no problem at all. On another trip, our truck broke down in the jungles of Costa Rica. We were stuck out in the middle of nowhere for 24 hours. Once again we had well-stocked backpacks, which saved the day. You can avoid serious problems. If you just plan things out wisely and are always prepared for the worst, you can go anywhere and have as much fun as anyone else.

WHAT THE DOC SAYS:

In addition to carrying extra food and diabetes supplies **with you at all times** while traveling, you have to adjust to time changes. Move meals back or forward a few hours at a time. If there is a large time difference, take extra short-acting insulin to cover highs and take your intermediate-acting insulin at the times you would normally take it—before breakfast, before dinner, or whenever, but use the time of your final destination. For example, if you are traveling from Chicago to London, you would take your pre-dinner insulin in Chicago, take short-acting insulin while flying, and take a pre-breakfast intermediate-acting insulin on London time. For an insulin pump, you just have to give your boluses before eating.

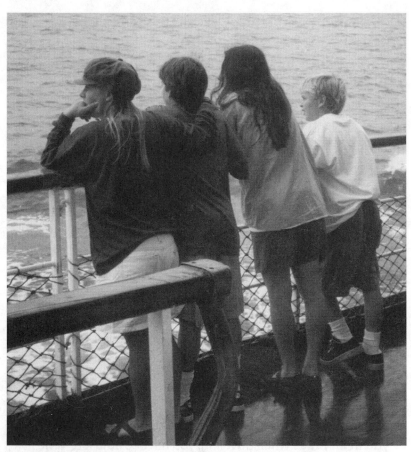

Jenny, Spike, Mary, and Bo, cruising in the Galapagos

THE BACKPACK

This is what we carry in our backpacks when we travel. **Always keep your insulin and food with you in your backpack.**

The Main Body of the Backpack contains:

Insulin kit (page 11)   Snacks packed in
Meter kit   brown paper bags
Gatorade   Jacket
1 box crackers   Hat

1 box cookies   Book
Jerky

The Side Pocket contains:

Glucagon kit   Ketostix
Frosting   Tylenol
Imodium—for diarrhea   Neosporin
Compazine, Phenergan,
    or Tigan—for nausea
    (Compazine is not for children)

The Inside Pocket contains:

Passport   Money
Tickets

The Large Front Pocket contains:

Toothbrush   Special medical
Chapstick   supplies, for
Deodorant   example, asthma
Razor   medication
Swimmer's Ear drops or   Pens
    ear plugs   Small notebook
Sunscreen lotion

WHAT THE DOC SAYS:

Always carry some form of identification stating that you
have diabetes and an instruction sheet on what to do if you
can't help yourself, for example, how to use the cake frosting or the glucagon.

THE FULL MEDICAL KIT

When we go on a big trip, say surfing to Costa Rica, we carry a Full Medical Kit. Ours contains:

First aid cream and first aid guide

Benadryl—for allergy

Antiseptic spray

Ibuprofen—for pain and inflammation

Meclizine—for motion sickness

Band-Aids

Rolled tourniquet

Tweezers

Antiseptic cream— for cuts

Cold sore cream

Instant ice pack

Swimmer's Ear drops— preventative

Bee sting kit

Gauze pads

Scissors

Needle and thread

Prescription Drugs

We also carry:

Glucagon kit

Hydrocortisone cream—anti-inflammatory, for rashes

Antipyrine/Benzocaine Otic—for ear pain

Cortisporin Otic—for pain, infection, inflammation

Imodium or Lomotil—anti-diarrhea, can be taken up to 4 times a day

Compazine or Phenergan—anti-nausea

Keflex—for upper respiratory infection, skin abrasions

Tobrex—for eye infection

Vicodin—for stingray or jellyfish stings. Immerse stingray wound in hot water, as hot as you can stand, to neutralize the toxin. Ammonia can also neutralize the acid in the toxin, so you might carry a small bottle. When you are out in the boonies, put urine on a jellyfish sting.

WHAT THE DOC SAYS:

You can carry different brands of medical supplies in your backpack, just be sure that they do what you expect them to do. For example, Neosporin Plus is an antibiotic cream to keep cuts from getting infected. Talk with your doctor about which drugs—both over-the-counter and prescription drugs—you might want to carry with you.

9

Driving

I have never personally experienced any real lows or scary incidents while driving. However, I realize that the potential for accidents as a result of an insulin reaction is real, and so I take all the necessary precautions. I'd like to think that it is my wariness that has kept things running smoothly.

Driving comes with added freedoms and added responsibilities.

- **Never drive with low blood sugar**. If you drive while very low, you might as well be driving drunk. You will be sluggish, slow to react, and simply asking for trouble. Instead, either get a friend to drive you to a food source or eat some of the food you have in your vehicle and wait until it takes effect before you drive anywhere.
- **Keep a refrigeration device (or cooler) in your vehicle**. I have an electric cooler that plugs into my cigarette lighter. There is plenty of room for my kit, extra insulin, and food such as Gatorade, granola bars, peanuts, jerky, and anything else I may feel like eating. This is the single greatest benefit of always having my truck around—independence from

always carrying lots of food on my person and always trying to find a refrigerator.

▪ **Don't worry about leaving a social event momentarily to get food.** If mealtime rolls around and you need to eat, now you can go get food whenever you like. Having your own vehicle makes your life a little more private. You no longer have to plan out your whole day or make a fuss over needing to eat. I still recommend telling people where you are going, in case you're lower than you think and you end up needing someone to come looking for you.

▪ **Don't be afraid to pull off the road if you are not feeling right**. Pull over, have a drink of Gatorade, test your sugar, and either shoot up or eat depending on your level. This is what emergency-only stopping places are for.

▪ **Be extra prepared on long drives.** When I drive home from college, I'm on the road for at least 5 or 6 hours. I always keep a bottle of Gatorade, several granola bars, and a big bag of chips on the seat next to me in case I start feeling low between fast food stops. I also keep jerky there, so I can have a low-carb snack if I get hungry.

▪ **Carry a card in your wallet that identifies you as a diabetic.** Keep it right next to your license. This way if you get pulled over for suspected drunken driving (which may happen if you don't realize that you are low), the officer will realize that you need sugar and possibly further medical attention. Also, if you are in an accident, the paramedics will know that you need special attention.

▪ **Wear a medical ID bracelet or necklace.**

Driving gives everyone tremendous freedom, especially diabetics. No longer must you carry a cooler—you can keep one in your car. No longer must you worry constantly about getting an ice pack—you can have a mobile refrigeration unit. No longer must you worry about where your next meal will come from—you can drive down the block to a fast food place or store. As long as you are a bit more responsible and never get behind the wheel when you are low, being able to drive can help make your diabetes an even smaller inconvenience.

WHAT THE DOC SAYS:

Never get into a car, either as a driver or a passenger, when you feel low. Always eat or drink a rapid-acting sugar food and then eat a longer-acting snack. Check your sugar before beginning to drive and don't drive until your blood sugar is at least 80–100 mg/dl. If driving alone, make sure that you have a rapid-acting sugar food or drink and a snack on the seat next to you, so you can reach them easily. Most important of all, don't wait to eat when you feel low. Stop the car right away, eat, and don't start driving again until your blood sugar is in the safe range. As you do in treating all lows, drink a juice box or take cake frosting or glucose tablets to raise your blood sugar levels rapidly, and then eat a granola bar or half a sandwich—food with carbohydrates and protein in it.

Remember to wear a medical ID bracelet or necklace when driving. This will increase the likelihood that you will be appropriately treated with glucose if you get low. This also will help you avoid being mistakenly charged with "driving under the influence" (DUI).

10

Partying

When you get into your mid-teens, chances are that you'll be invited to some parties and chances are that not all of them will be alcohol and drug free. You have to be especially careful with drugs of any kind. And, when you choose not to use them, having diabetes is a perfect excuse to use against peer pressure. I have found that my friends respect my wishes when I tell them I am not going to drink because of diabetes—I am sure yours will, too.

Here's what to do at a party:

■ **Don't drink much at all.** You really shouldn't drink alcohol at all, but if you do, only drink a little. Some alcoholic beverages are full of sugar, so a beer is like drinking a regular Coke. This will cause your sugar to rise and then fall rapidly when it wears off. If you do drink, be sure to eat as well, so you have something to stabilize your sugar. Never drink enough to get drunk and pass out. This is the worst possible scenario. If you pass out and forget to eat or even forget to shoot up, you are asking for trouble.

- **Tell your friends to watch out for you**. If you are drinking, make sure someone knows what to do if you pass out, such as give you sugar and call your mom and dad immediately.
- **Don't use tobacco**. Nicotine causes problems with the tiny blood vessels in your arms and legs and diabetes does that, too. Smoking for even a short period of time damages your circulation, and you want to keep your blood vessels healthy all the time. Who wants to smoke anyway?
- **Be a designated driver**. I drive my friends around and stay completely sober at parties 95% of the time. This is another good way to handle peer pressure. It's always fun to be sober and laugh at all your friends anyway.
- **Whatever you choose to do, do it in moderation**. If you drink, don't drink a six-pack. If you smoke (I don't know why you would want to), only smoke a cigarette or two at parties and nowhere else. If you try marijuana, only take a couple of hits. The munchies can get you into trouble, but if you pass out and don't eat at all, you will get into worse trouble.
- **Don't be afraid to call mom and dad and tell them that you aren't feeling well.** This is a good idea for anyone, but it is truly important for diabetics.

You have to know your limits. Getting addicted to any of these substances will lead to extremely serious consequences for you, and it truly isn't worth it. Just remember that if you choose to try one of these substances, you must eat, too. A high blood sugar is much better than a low one. However, if you choose to avoid these things altogether, diabetes offers you the perfect reason.

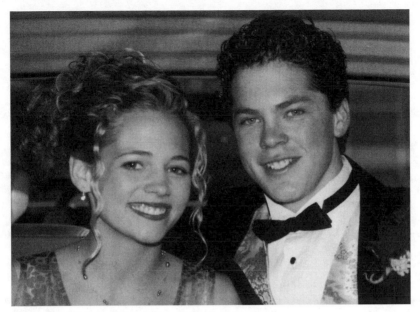

Krystal and Spike going to the prom

WHAT THE DOC SAYS:

Although you may be tired of hearing adults telling you to "Just say no," you need to know that cigarettes, alcohol, and drugs do pose definite serious risks if you have diabetes, over and above the risks they pose for nondiabetic people. Spike and Bo give balanced, responsible, and realistic guidelines for you to use in those situations where you may find yourself tempted by these substances. Know the facts, and know the risks that you face, particularly on account of your diabetes. The biggest risk from the diabetes perspective is that an altered mental state due to alcohol or drugs can cause you to miss the warning signs of low blood sugar,

continued

which may result in a seizure or coma. Also, alcohol can cause low blood sugar, especially if you don't eat while you drink. Cigarettes add to the risk of heart attacks, strokes, and other disorders for which diabetes already increases the risk, as well as increase the risk of eye and kidney complications. We all know these substances have the risk of addiction and bad effects on overall health in the long run. Be smart. Use your head and save your heart for better things.

11

Starting College

I recently graduated from Stanford University. Diabetes didn't affect me any differently at college than it did at high school, but before entering college, I made some special arrangements. Housing plans and meal plans are two parts of college life that need your particular attention.

Here's what to do during the enrollment process:

■ **Mark the "handicapped" or "chronically ill" box on your applications**. This will let the school know that you have a condition that requires special attention, and this will start the process.

■ **Register at the disabilities office**. Diabetes isn't truly a disability, as it can't keep you from doing a single thing; but registering will allow you to get special housing and meal plans. These aren't totally necessary, but they will make your life much easier.

■ **Get housing that has a kitchen or is near 24-hour food**. Either get a dorm with a late-night cafeteria or housing that is near fast-food places or eating clubs on campus. You never know when you will have a late-night low. You will need at least a small snack after each late-night study session, so there is no point in making it hard on yourself and having to walk miles to get food.

- **Keep a drawer stocked with food in your room.**
- **Put a small refrigerator in your dorm room.** I don't recommend this as a substitute for housing near food but as a complement to it. At school I snacked out of my refrigerator almost nightly to keep my sugars up, and I don't know what I would do without one.
- **Get a meal plan that has no absolute limit.** The college has to offer you as much food as you need, and you really should get a plan that allows this, even if you have to pay extra.
- **Take any advantages that come your way.** At many schools, if you are registered as a diabetic, they will have someone take notes for you at any class you miss for medical reasons. They also must allow you to make up any tests missed for that reason. Some schools may even have affirmative action programs for chronically ill students. I don't really like to take handouts, but diabetes has made my life a little bit harder, and I have had to work harder to get where I am today, so I welcome anything that makes it a little bit easier.

I am fortunate the university that I am attending, Stanford, offers all of these things. Some schools may not be able to offer these benefits because of limited resources, so be sure to look into what is available when you're making decisions. Letting as many offices and people at college know of my condition has made the transition from living at home to living on my own as smooth as it was for everyone else.

Note: Our mom's book, *Real Life Parenting of Kids With Diabetes*, devotes a chapter to going off to college with lots of lists to make your transition easier.

12

Dealing with Doctors

Getting a good doctor or two is vital when you have diabetes, as you may tend to need a few more visits a year than others. The twice-a-year major blood work visits are important, too. They can really tell your doctor a lot and help you to keep tight control. However, one big thing with doctors is that they want what is absolutely the healthiest option for you, and this often conflicts with what you may want to do. There is generally a middle ground that will still keep you very healthy.

Some things to do to stay healthy:

▪ **Get a specialist**. Endocrinologists and others who specialize in the treatment of diabetes are a key to living healthy. They know things that no general practitioner would dream of, and they can often explain the processes of diabetes in understandable ways. Having an idea of what is going on in your body really helps you control it. Besides, it's no fun to tell people "I don't know" when they ask you what diabetes really is.

■ **Try to find a pediatrician or general practitioner with at least some background in diabetes.** Specialists are expensive and, chances are, you will only visit them a few times a year and only for diabetes-related issues and diabetic check-ups. The doctor who takes care of you all the rest of the time should know how different medications and ailments affect hormones and blood sugars. However, don't be afraid to call your specialist whenever you have any type of question.

■ **Don't worry if you don't follow your doctor's orders exactly.** The doctors will tell you never to eat sugar and always to get so many minutes of exercise each day and to eat only so many calories at such and such times a day. Their advice is sound, and following it will keep you the healthiest but probably not the happiest. A piece of cake (a small piece) at a birthday party isn't bad. A day where you just sit on the couch (once in awhile) is all right. Eating a little more when you are hungry is OK too. Diabetes doesn't have to keep you from being a kid and having fun.

We had an ice cream party in my fifth grade class about a week after I had been in for a major diabetic check-up. I turned down all offers of ice cream and just sat outside and pitied myself. That is no way to live. It's perfectly fine to live it up a little and "cheat" a little (as long as it doesn't become a habit). I should have checked my blood sugar and taken enough insulin to counteract a small bowl of ice cream and then eaten some. Don't misunderstand me here—it is extremely important to visit your specialist regularly and take what they have to say seriously. But it is also extremely important to enjoy your life.

WHAT THE DOC SAYS:

I couldn't agree more! This topic brings up the issue of freedom versus responsibility, which is, I believe, the core of the
"diabetic struggle" in the teenage years. Remember: you
can usually have both. I never use the word "cheat" when
referring to a change in the ideal self-care plan. There is
always a reason you don't follow your care plan to the letter, and it's important to look at it and recognize why, so
you can make self-care decisions that serve you best. Don't
be afraid to tell your doctor what is important to you. If you
respect yourself and your desires and speak up, your doctor
can usually find a way to work with you to maintain good
glucose control in most situations. For example, most physi-
cians no longer prohibit desserts but teach you how to
incorporate them into your meal plan. Remember, it is your
life you are talking about, and you are the expert on your
life. At the same time, the knowledge and experience of diabetes professionals, parents, and other adults important in
your life can also help you reach the goals you set for yourself. Your doctor and other diabetes care professionals are
your expert consultants, and they are there to best serve
your needs and interests.

13

When You Are Sick

If you are not feeling good, it's not always because of your blood sugar or because of your diabetes acting up. Diabetics get sick, too. So it's not a bad idea to check your blood sugar, and try to figure out what's going on. **Whenever you are feeling down, that's the first thing you should do—check your sugar.**

When you're sick, your blood sugar tends to run a little high. On top of being sick, high sugar makes you feel worse. Test your sugar often; you might need some extra short-acting insulin shots throughout the day. When I'm high, I take extra shots of 2 or 3 units of Regular, drink lots of water, and check for ketones.

SICK-DAY PLAN

Make sure your doctor OKs your sick day regimen. Here's mine:

▌ **Nausea: When you are nauseated, the rules change.** Now there is the possibility of vomiting up your food, so you might want to drastically reduce the amount of insulin you take at any one time. Sometimes my doctor might have me stop taking long-lasting insulin for a day or two and take short-acting insulin every 4–6 hours. I drink lots of fluids with calories in them. For instance, when I get sick, I drink Gatorade and real 7-Up and eat plain white toast. I also like to have popsicles around because they are good and easy to eat. It's not usually a good idea to eat sugar, but when you're nauseated, you need the calories.

- **Vomiting: If you vomit more than once, it's time to call your doctor.** You'll need a prescription drug for the nausea. (We have a prescription for Compazine we keep at home and take with us when we travel.) You will need help. Mom or dad should always stay home with you when you are nauseous or vomiting!

- **Compazine: Knocks you out.** Somebody must be home with you when you use it.

- **TLC: When you are sick, you need attention.** You need somebody to help you with all the blood testing and drinking. You need to keep your mind busy by watching TV or playing video games or the computer. A back rub is always nice.

When you're sick, you'll probably be talking with your doctor. Don't get bummed out. Just remember, you'll get over it.

SUPPLIES TO KEEP ON HAND FOR SICK DAYS

Real 7-Up	Gatorade	Frosting
Sugar popsicles	Plain white bread	Suckers
Chicken soup	Saltine crackers	Candy

Liquids in very small amounts go down the best, then I add Saltines and white bread.

KETONES

This is how we handle ketones:

- **When do you develop ketones?** Sometimes when you have had high blood sugar for several hours, you feel sick all over. Your body is achy, you feel sluggish, and you may have developed ketones. You should always have ketone strips around the house. Test for ketones when you're sick or when your blood sugar is running high. It's a simple urine test.
- **Ketone sticks.** After you dip the ketone stick in your urine, in a matter of seconds the stick turns colors. If dark purple shows up, you are making lots of ketones. Don't panic. You

can get rid of ketones in a few hours. When I see high ketones on a ketone strip, I take a couple of extra units of Regular insulin (short-acting) and drink a lot of water. I test for ketones every hour, watching the color on the strip fade until I'm back to normal.

- **Getting rid of ketones.** Spike and I look at testing for ketones as a positive thing. It's just another way to help you keep your blood sugars normal, between 80 and 140 mg/dl. Lots of ketones means your body is burning fat and you may have had high blood sugar for several hours. When ketones show up, we work on getting rid of them right away. The first time you have high ketones you'll probably call your doctor. After that you'll know what to do: test, take a couple of extra units of short-acting insulin, eat a bite of food, relax, and drink lots of water. (We always eat a little when we inject insulin.) After an hour passes, test, and if ketones are still high, inject again and drink some more. Keep doing this until the ketones are gone. It may take only one session but sometimes it takes three or four.
- **Ketones and vomiting.** If you are sick and vomiting and have ketones, it's time to call the doctor!

Note: I never take more than 2 extra units of Regular insulin late at night. I don't want to crash. (Crash is what we call what happens when your blood sugar gets really low, and you feel shaky, weak, and maybe emotional.)

WHAT THE DOC SAYS:

Ketones are acids that are produced when your body breaks down fat. If you have high blood sugar, too, ketones mean that you do not have enough insulin in your body to

---

keep fat from breaking down. Your body gets rid of ketones in your urine, so it is important to drink lots of fluids if ketones are present. If ketones are produced more quickly than your kidneys can get rid of them, they will accumulate in your blood and cause nausea and vomiting. It is important to try to get rid of ketones before you get to this point because nausea and vomiting can lead to dehydration and acidosis (too much acid in your blood). This can result in a vicious cycle in which vomiting leads to dehydration, which makes the ketoacidosis worse, which, in turn, causes more vomiting. At this point, you often need to be hospitalized and treated with intravenous (IV) fluids and insulin to break the cycle. The only way to keep ketones from forming is to take extra insulin.

Some people are very sensitive to insulin and only take small doses, but others are taking much larger doses. The dose of short-acting insulin that you will take to treat your ketones depends on your daily insulin dose. You should talk to your doctor or diabetes educator to determine the correct dose for you.

Accidents or Surgery

14

One morning while skateboarding to class, I had a little accident. Maneuvering through heavy student traffic, I hit a little bump in the road and my skateboard decided to stop. The only problem was that I kept going. I made a perfect landing on my left elbow, immediately picked myself up, and went on to class. Five days later I was in for orthopedic surgery.

When you go in for surgery, you never know exactly what's going to happen. For instance, the doc told me he was going to put a pair of pins in my arm and I would be out of surgery and back in my dorm room to study for finals in just a few short hours. As it turned out, the pins didn't work, so they went for the 6-inch steel plate option and an operation that took about 4½ hours and left me on morphine for 3 days. I was too doped up to take my finals, but I certainly learned a bit about dealing with diabetes while laid up in the hospital.

When you are going in for surgery:

■ **Be in charge of your own insulin**. (You'll need your mom or dad on the job.)
■ **Take your kits.** See page 11.
■ **Inform everyone you meet before, during, and after surgery that you have diabetes.**

- **Expect to use frequent small doses of insulin**. I took 2 units of Regular insulin every few hours for the first 2 days.
- **Double check the doses when nurses are giving you your insulin**. (A cc is not the same as an insulin unit.) Many nurses are not used to the very small unit measurements on an insulin syringe. You must check what they want to give you, every time. If you don't agree, discuss it. Ask questions!

I'm going to outline what happened to me, so you will know what to expect if you have a snowboard or skateboard accident or other debilitating injury that requires surgery. Your doctor will be in charge, and the hospital will have a diabetes protocol. **Nevertheless, you are the one who knows the most about how to handle your own diabetes**. You're the expert on you.

- **The night before surgery**: I ate like a king—steak, baked potatoes, the works!
- **The morning of surgery**: No insulin, no food, no water.
- **During surgery**: My mother was there in the hospital, standing by. (Have someone with you.)
- **Post-surgery**: The recovery team did frequent blood sugar tests.
- **Post-surgery insulin**: The first insulin I received was 3 units of short-acting insulin at 3 PM that afternoon.

(I was groggy and then on morphine for 2 days. My mom monitored my blood sugar and discussed every injection with the nursing staff. We were surprised at how little insulin I needed to take those first 2 days. It made sense though. I was eating almost nothing.)

- **Nausea**: When coming out of the anesthesia, I needed something for nausea. Once the nausea was handled, I ate a little. Then it was determined how much insulin I should take. Again, only 2 or 3 units of short-acting insulin.
- **Post-surgery day 2**: Frequent blood sugar tests. Frequent small doses of short-acting insulin. I didn't take any long-acting insulin until day 3.
- **Post-surgery day 3**: I returned to my dorm but was on heavy pain medication, Vicodin. We discovered that I was pretty out of it and needed help monitoring my diabetes, so I went home for a few days where my "support team" could take care of me.

Note: In the hospital and post surgery, you will need someone with you to help you handle your diabetes!

WHAT THE DOC SAYS:

The overall point here is a good one—nobody knows your body and diabetes better than you, and you should take an active role in your hospital management. However, situations such as those described here can be very complex. You will find it to your advantage to work with the members of your health care team in charge of your hospital care, since their medical knowledge will be most important to you at this stressful time. Balance is the key. While you don't want to get into power struggles with your hospital nurses or doctors over every insulin dose, you may at times need to assert that you are the expert on you, and they should respect your knowledge of your body and your diabetes.

15

Insulin, Pumps, and Support

TWO KINDS OF INSULIN—ONE SYRINGE

When you get used to using insulin 3, 4, or 5 times a day, you can forget what you have just done, so having a routine is important. This is the routine I follow. When it is time for an injection, this is what I do:

▌ Take two bottles of insulin out of the fridge and put them on the kitchen counter. I work from left to right, so I always put the Regular insulin on the left. I put the NPH insulin on the right. Then I double-check the bottles to make sure they are two different kinds of insulin.

▌ I always draw the Regular (short-acting) first, which is the smaller amount. Then I follow by drawing the NPH.

TWO KINDS OF INSULIN—TWO SYRINGES

In our teen years, we changed from NPH long-lasting insulin to Ultralente. Ultralente (U) cannot be mixed with Regular

(R) insulin. With two bottles and two shots, you can get mixed up. To avoid using the same bottle twice (which equals a bad overdose, if it's two shots of Regular) we came up with the following system.

■ Take two bottles of insulin out of the fridge. Put them on the kitchen counter—R on the left, U on the right.
■ Put a needle in each bottle. Just leave them there sticking out.
■ Draw the needed amount of R and inject.
■ The second injection of insulin will be from the other bottle. The syringe is still in the bottle of U, so there is no mistake about which one to use.

We figured out this system after a couple of accidental overdoses. **If you should inject with two doses of Regular insulin, call your doctor immediately. Tell your mom and dad. You will need help getting through the next 8 hours, but you can do it.** Both Spike and I have each accidentally overdosed on Regular. For the next 8 hours, we tested every half hour, and we ate huge amounts of high-calorie food (Gatorade, candy bars, ice cream, bread, whatever we felt like).

Doctors prescribe different combinations of insulin. You might be taking short-acting Humalog and long-acting NPH, or short-acting Regular and long-acting NPH, or short-acting Regular and long-acting Ultralente. Whatever the combination you use, the rules are the same.

Note: Spike and I let our mom and dad draw the insulin and give the injections until we were teenagers. It was nice for us not to have to take on complete responsibility until we wanted to.

THE INSULIN PUMP

Since Spike and I have no personal experience with the insulin pump, we asked two girls from our playgroup, Kids with Diabetes, Inc., about their new insulin pumps. Vanessa and Kelly say they love their pumps and would not go back to insulin injections. They said it took a few days to get comfortable sleeping with the pump and they had to get used to changing their clothes with the tubing connected to their bodies.

Kelly, age 13, finds the pump more convenient, giving her more independence and freedom. Vanessa, age 12, added that she had better control and felt better wearing her pump. They gave us some details about preparing to wear an insulin pump.

Getting Started

For 2 weeks the girls worked with an instructor who showed them a video and explained how to use the pump and answered all their questions. Then they were fitted with pumps. The nurse plugged in the pumps by injecting a small, short needle with a tiny flexible tube inside, called a cannula, into their sides. The needle is pulled out and the cannula stays under your skin. At first it is a little tricky to learn to do this yourself. There is a connection that sits right on the surface of the skin. The part that sticks out is about the size of an insulin bottle cap, and very thin tubing, about 30 inches long, goes from that connection to the pump.

During the first few days, their pumps were full of saline solution. They took before-meal blood tests and dialed in the correct amount of insulin. The computer chip in the pump kept records for their doctor to review. They practiced "suspending" the pump in order to stop it from delivering insulin. (To do this, you scroll down on the menu and click the suspend mode. Once it is suspended, the pump beeps every 15 minutes to let you know that it has stopped delivering insulin.) If they ever got low, they needed to know how to stop the flow of insulin. The pump could also be disconnected from the body by simply unsnapping the tubing. There is a one-way gasket that does not allow insulin to leak out. They practiced unsnapping the tubing from the infusion site and putting their pumps on the suspend mode.

For those first two weeks, they took lots of blood tests every few hours. That's so their doctors could get a baseline. They practiced wearing the pump, changing clothes, and showering with it. To shower, they unsnap the tubing from the connection at the skin and shower. There is no need to cover up the site because the gasket keeps out the water. While showering, they store the pump and tubing in a plastic bag to keep them clean and dry.

Once a baseline was established, the saline solution was replaced with Humalog insulin, and they were ready to go!

The playgroup kids asked all kinds of questions. Vanessa explained that she changed the infusion site every 3 days. She said it was hard to inject the tiny needle the first time, but that she had gotten used to it, and now it was no big deal to do. Both Vanessa and Kelly showed the kids their pumps and the tubing and the infusion site on their sides where the tubing meets the tiny top of the cannula.

Kelly explained why the pump gives such good control. The pump is programmed to release a steady amount of Humalog

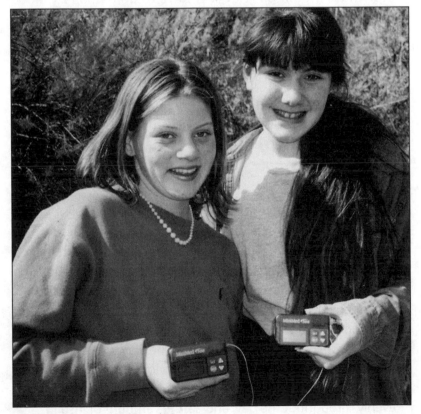

Playgroup pumpers Kelly and Vanessa

insulin into your system. (The constant stream of insulin is determined by your baseline.) Then at snack time and meal-time, you do a blood test and look at what you are about to eat, figure the right amount of insulin, and dial it in.

They said the pump costs about $5,000, but their insurance paid for most of it.

Safety Tip

When the girls go on field trips or camping trips, they carry a kit of extra insulin and syringes, just in case there is a malfunc-tion with their pumps. They still have to do five or six blood tests a day but no more shots!

Spike and I looked into the pump several years ago. We were playing contact sports and surfing every day, so the pump wasn't right for our lifestyle. With the improvements in the pump since then, Spike and I have both gone on the pump and truly enjoy the flexibility and diabetes control it provides.

WHAT THE DOC SAYS:

When you want to keep your blood sugar levels closer to normal, you get into what is called intensive diabetes man-agement. It's a three-part approach: nutrition, insulin, and exercise. You use carb counting or meal planning so you can predict the effect the food you eat will have on your blood sugar and insulin needs. You use multiple daily injec-tions of insulin or the pump to mimic the way your body provides insulin throughout the day to lower blood sugar. The pump supplies a **basal** amount of insulin slowly and evenly throughout the day, and a **bolus** amount of insulin

---

whenever you eat food. Exercise helps keep your body fit and improves the way your muscles use blood sugar.

You will need to check your blood sugar more often to learn how it reacts to different foods, insulin levels, and levels of exercise. You keep a written log of the foods you eat, the insulin you take, the exercise you get, the stress you're under, and your blood sugar levels. This helps you figure out your own patterns, so you can make decisions and changes in your self-care plan.

Some of the advantages of an intensive care plan are:

1. being able to keep your blood sugar closer to normal, so you feel better
2. giving yourself the best chance for avoiding complications later in life
3. having more flexibility about when you eat and how much you eat
4. improving your health and fitness

Some of the difficulties of an intensive care plan are:

1. needing detailed diabetes education
2. increasing your risk of having hypoglycemia
3. needing motivation to keep doing all you have to do
4. increasing the cost of maintaining your diabetes in supplies, office visits, etc.

Intensive regimens are flexible regimens because they get you out of the "2 shots a day, have to eat right now!" mentality of diabetes care. If you have any interest at all in trying out the flexible regimen, talk with your doctor or diabetes educator.

SUPPORT GROUPS

You've heard us mention our playgroup, Kids with Diabetes, Inc. We found that it is very important to meet with other kids who have diabetes and to share stories and experiences and ideas about what to do. We recruit kids who are newly diagnosed to come to our playgroup and offer them a helping hand. In fact, that is why we wrote this book—to offer support to all other kids with diabetes. Our mom offers the same kind of support to the parents, and we all help each other. Support is very important if you are going to live well with diabetes.

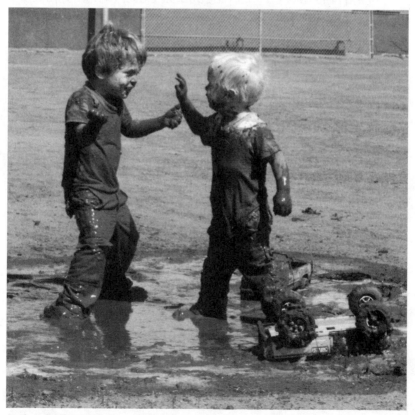

Spike and Bo, in their natural element

WHAT THE DOC SAYS:

I strongly recommend that you consider finding and joining a diabetes support group for kids or teens. The teenage years are hard enough without having to deal with diabetes. Having a group of people your age to meet with on a regular basis can provide you with the type of support you need to stay motivated to take care of yourself. We know the benefits of support groups for young people with diabetes, including improved diabetes knowledge, self-care, and communication with parents. Let's face it, we human beings are social animals. We all need some help, guidance, and advice sometimes, and we all need to **give** some help and guidance, too. You will benefit more ways than you realize now. To find a group in your area, talk to your health care team, local ADA chapter, or other local diabetes organizations.

Food—Short, Medium, and Long

16

When we were little, we made up this idea of putting all foods into categories—short, medium, and long. Short means that the sugar in the food gets into your system quickly. Medium foods take about 15 minutes to kick in, and long foods digest very slowly over a period of a couple of hours.

- **Short**: All things with sugar, candy bars, granola bars, cookies, milk, ice cream and cake, Gatorade, fruit juice, slushies, and smoothies are short. They contain sugar, which is a carbohydrate.
- **Medium**: Starchy things like bread, pasta, rice, chips, and crackers are medium. Starch is also a carbohydrate.
- **Long**: High-protein items like meat, chicken, fish, cheese, cottage cheese, eggs, and nuts are long.

HANDY CATEGORIES

It's really handy to have food in these three categories. When you are little, it's a lot easier to understand medium than it is to understand carbohydrate. Since we had to eat every 2 hours, we used short, medium, and long in our meal plans. As 6 year olds, we found it hard to remember that when you feel kind of down, you need a certain kind of food. It's easier to say, "I need a short," and somebody has it for you right there.

Friends

When you are young and your folks tell your neighbors about your food needs, it's easier for them and your friends' parents to think about food as short, medium, and long.

Backpack

Whenever you go anywhere, you need to have your backpack or your cooler with you packed with short, medium, and long foods.

Sports

When you are about ready to play sports, it's OK to have a little short.

TV

When you're watching TV, you should snack on long foods and maybe a little medium.

WHAT THE DOC SAYS:

All carbohydrates (short and medium foods) get converted to sugar. The body uses that sugar mainly for quick energy.

Proteins and fats (long foods) are more slowly absorbed and don't act as quickly as carbohydrates. The carbohydrates that are most quickly absorbed act most rapidly on your blood sugar. These are the simple sugars found in fruit juices, hard candies, glucose tablets, and cake frosting (short foods). Other carbohydrates need to be digested and broken down to simple sugars before they can act. These carbohydrates include granola bars, cookies, cake, bread, pasta, rice, chips, and crackers (medium foods). The more fat and protein there is in a food, the slower it is absorbed and the slower it acts on your blood sugar. High-protein foods, such as meat, chicken, cheese, eggs, and nuts (long foods) are good for long-lasting endurance activities.

Spike and Bo have a good system for deciding what to eat and when. For example, if you are doing a high-intensity exercise for only a little while, then a medium food should work well for you.

Besides cake frosting, honey is useful for treating low blood sugar. There are glucose gels available, too, but you may not like the taste of them. Jerky is a long food that Spike and Bo like, but other people may prefer peanut butter crackers or half of a turkey sandwich. Any (long) food with protein and fat will help keep your blood sugar on an even level once you have raised it by eating a short food.

WHAT WE LIKE TO EAT

Here is a list of some of the things we like to eat. We eat what we like; we just make sure we always have protein with carbohydrates. Our rule for meals and snacks: Never eat a carbohydrate alone.

Every morning our mom makes breakfast. By far our favorite is the breakfast burrito.

Breakfast

Breakfast Burrito	Another choice	Another choice
2 scrambled eggs	2 pieces bacon	Sausage
2 bacon or sausage	2 eggs scrambled	2 eggs
½ fried potato	in butter	½ fried potato or
Jack cheese	1 toast/butter	toast
In a warm flour	Grated cheese	½ glass whole milk
tortilla	½ glass whole milk	

We have a glass of water if we're high, ½ a glass of orange juice if we are low, or ½ a glass of whole milk if we're just right or starving. As we got older, the portions increased.

Snacks

When we were little, every morning our mom packed 3 separate snacks in 3 separate brown paper bags with the snack-time written on each: 10 AM, 12 noon, 2 PM. The bag went into the top of our coolers. It was a tight squeeze, but it made snacking easy.

10 AM	12 Noon	2 PM
String cheese	Trail mix	Cracker and cheese
Small banana	String cheese	Jerky
Crackers	Crackers	Grapes

Lunch

Our favorite lunch is a breakfast burrito. Other examples are:

Sandwich on low-carbohydrate bread
String cheese

Hamburger
Small banana

Hot dog
Small apple

Bacon, lettuce, and tomato sandwich

Pita bread stuffed with:
  Cream cheese
  Bacon pieces
  Cheddar cheese
  Lettuce

I used to take my mom's famous breakfast burritos to school for lunch. My friends started noticing that I had them every day. They tried them, and they really liked them. Pretty soon I was taking extra burritos to school everyday to share with my friends.

Soccer Games

If we had a soccer game after school, mom packed the following in our athletic bags:

1 box of crackers
1 small box of cookies

1 bag of beef jerky
1 large Gatorade

1 tube of frosting
$5.00

Dinner

When you have dinner, just combine your carbs with protein. If you are eating spaghetti, have a smaller helping of noodles with a big helping of meat sauce. When we are playing sports, we sometimes have spaghetti with a T-bone steak on the side.

Again, if we're high, we drink water with our meals. If we're low, we drink whole milk. Some examples of the dinners we eat are:

Steak	Chicken	Tacos
½ baked potato	Rice	Meat
Vegetable	Vegetable	Cheese
Salad	Salad	Lettuce
Cube steak	Stir fry	Spaghetti
Mashed potato	Chicken	Meat sauce
Gravy	Vegetables	Salad
Vegetable	Fried rice	Bread

Bedtime Snack

Always eat a bedtime snack. Combine a medium and a long food (a carb and a protein). Some good examples of this would be:

Toast with peanut butter
A second helping of dinner
Cereal, milk, and string cheese or peanuts
A tortilla with melted cheese

Because we play sports, we tend to eat pretty large bedtime snacks. You won't need so much food right before bed if you have had a quiet day. Never skip a bedtime snack. (If you go to bed, are about to fall off to sleep and remember you forgot your snack, get up and snack. That way you'll have a good night and a good morning.)

WHAT THE DOC SAYS:

When you're a teenager, eating well gives you the right amount of fuel, or calories, for normal growth and development and improves your overall health. In general, I usually recommend lots of fresh fruits and vegetables; whole grains; low-fat or fat-free milk; lean meats, poultry, and fish; healthy fats like nuts, avocado, and olive oil; and to the extent that your budget allows, organic foods free of pesticides and with no chemical processing. We all know that fast foods, high-fat sweets, or sugar-containing sodas taste good—I like to call them "play" foods. It makes common sense to eat these play foods only in moderation because they give you very little nutritional benefit for all the calories they also give you.

Remember that even though there is no such thing as a "bad" or "forbidden" food, when you add sweets to your meal plan, it's important to trade them gram for gram for the other carbohydrates you would normally eat, so you don't get high blood sugars or gain weight. Your dietitian can help you develop a meal plan to fit you and your lifestyle at the age you are right now. The meal plan will need to be changed as you grow, add sports or new activities, or want to try different foods.

WHAT ARE PROTEINS AND CARBS?

Remember short, medium, and long? Each meal should contain protein, carbohydrates, fat, and vegetables. Here we give you a list of food to keep in the house, so you can have good stuff to eat without making your blood sugars go wild.

Food to Have Around the House

Short: Sugars (Fast carbohydrates)	Medium: Carbohydrates	Long: Protein
Fruit juices	Cake	Beef
Candy	Cookies	Bacon
Milk	Crackers	Chicken
Frosting	Chips	Sausage
Glucose tablets	Fruits	Cheese
	Potatoes	Cottage cheese
	Pasta	String cheese
	Rice	Eggs
	Cereal	Hamburger
	Beans	Ham
	Whole milk	Fish
		Peanut butter
		Turkey
		Tuna
		Hot dogs

Our Rules

- Never eat a carbohydrate alone.
- Fill the house with proteins for snacks.
- Have sugar foods around for when you are low.

WHAT THE DOC SAYS:

For you science buffs, here's some extra detail you might find interesting. While both proteins and carbohydrates contain approximately 4 calories per gram, they serve very dif-

---

ferent purposes in our bodies. Proteins are for structure and action. For instance, the solid mass of our muscles is mainly protein, as are the enzymes needed for many important biochemical processes. Carbohydrates, on the other hand, primarily provide the energy our bodies need to function.

It is mostly the carbohydrate that you eat that raises your blood sugar, so as far as blood sugar goes, the amount of carbs in the meal is the most important number. If you figure out how many grams of carbohydrate you eat in a meal, you can match it with the right amount of insulin to bring your blood sugar back to normal. Counting carbs offers you a huge amount of freedom and flexibility in your daily life, as you decide what to eat and adjust your insulin accordingly. If you need more information on carb counting and how it can benefit you, consult your registered dietitian (RD) or certified diabetes educator (CDE).

17

What Everyone Needs to Know— So They Can Help

Your parents can copy the three documents in this chapter and substitute the important information about you. Give the three documents to every teacher, principal, and coach you meet. Give a copy to your friends' parents, too.

1. **Symptoms: Stick a copy of symptoms in the top of your cooler.** This way if you crash, people will know what to do. This page gives clear directions for what needs to be done when you suffer a low blood sugar—when you crash.

2. **Why diabetics need extra calories: This explains why you eat so often.** It's a lot easier when your teachers and coaches are aware of how often you need to eat. First of all, they won't hassle you, and second, they will be more supportive.

3. **Schedule: This page describes what you do every day.** When those in authority see on paper how hard you try to maintain normal blood sugars, they tend to be helpful and understanding when you need to reschedule a test or are late for school.

SYMPTOMS

(This is what works for us. Replace my name with yours and list your specific symptoms. Give this to all teachers, coaches, parents, and close friends.)

When Bo Shows These Symptoms

Symptoms	Mild	Headache
		Stomachache
	Serious	Feels empty
		Shaky hands
		Feels faint
	Extreme	Very upset, crying, angry

Do this

    1st: Give fruit drink (Gatorade) from backpack
    2nd: Follow with granola bar, crackers, then jerky
         (He should feel better in 3–5 minutes)

■ **Your Role**: These symptoms are listed in the order they usually appear. If you are with Bo while he is feeling empty and is shaky, crying or upset, then you need to open the juice can or Gatorade, put it into his hands and **make sure** he drinks it. Hand him the opened granola bar and **make sure** he eats it.

■ **Why?** These symptoms occur because his blood sugar is dangerously low. He is about to pass out. At this point his thinking is cloudy, he cannot function, and he needs sugar!

■ **Call**: If you see the more serious symptoms after giving a sugar drink, give more sugar drink. In about 10 minutes, follow with cookies, milk (short), crackers, chips (medium), and jerky (long). Then call Virginia (mom) or Rick (dad).

Extreme Emergency

If Bo should pass out: **Open frosting in backpack immediately.**

Squirt all of it into the corner of his mouth between cheek and gums.

If no frosting is available, put sugar in the corner of his mouth between cheek and gums. As soon as he is alert enough to swallow, follow with a fruit drink, real Coke, or Gatorade. Call Virginia, call Rick. If no luck, call 911 or go to a hospital. Tell them he is suffering from low blood sugar, which is insulin shock, and he needs glucose.

Mom's phone numbers

Home:_____ Car:_____ Business:_____ Beeper:_____

Dad's phone numbers

Home:_____ Car:_____ Business:_____ Beeper:_____

Doctor's phone number_____

Office: _____   Emergency number: _____

Hospital phone number: _____

Note: Have a "Permission to Treat" document on file at your local hospital and at your school.

WHY DIABETICS NEED EXTRA CALORIES

(This explanation about why you need extra calories should come from your folks. It gives teachers and coaches an understanding of what is going on with your body and how they can help.)

Maintaining normal blood sugar in a growing kid requires an absolute constant flow of calories into the system. Bo must be allowed to eat the moment he senses his blood sugar is low or dropping, in addition to his scheduled snacks.

- **Bo**: Eats when he feels low.
  Must eat every 2 hours.
  Needs more calories when he exercises and takes tests.
- **Help**: Bo doesn't always feel a low coming on. If you notice odd behavior, ask him if he needs calories.
- **Vomiting**: Requires immediate calories, liquids, and care at home.
- **Injury**: Can make blood sugar soar, then fall. If injured, call Virginia (mom). She will come down and do some tests.
- **Blood Tests**: Bo will need to do blood tests at school sometimes. All the kids know about these tests. Do not send Bo off alone for a blood test. He is probably testing his blood because he is feeling low, and he may need some help to test and eat.
- **Call Home**: Bo needs to call home when he feels odd or bad. First have him snack. Then have a student walk to the office with him. Low sugar can cause him to become disoriented.
- **Understanding**: Teachers should not humiliate Bo about his calorie needs.
- **Vigilance**: Bo plays all-star soccer, surfs, and snowboards. He can do anything. We simply must be vigilant EVERY TIME.

The important concept here is not so much extra calories, as "getting what he needs when he needs them" calories. A teenager with diabetes does not actually need any more calories than a teenager without diabetes, but he or she does need free access to food at all times in case of an unexpected low blood sugar. Unfortunately, this need can conflict with the rules and schedules of your school or other programs. It is very important that you talk about this special need with those people in charge to avoid unnecessary, frustrating, and possibly dangerous conflicts when you feel low between scheduled meals and need to eat a snack. The general principle appears in this book again and again—plan ahead so you can set up a situation around you that allows you the freedom you need to care for your diabetes.

YOUR SCHEDULE

(When adults get this schedule, it helps them understand you and diabetes. Then they can help.)

6:30 AM	Blood test
	Insulin injection Regular and NPH
	(You might be using Humalog and NPH)
	Breakfast
8:30 AM	Snack—NPH (long-lasting insulin) kicks in
10:30 AM	Snack

12:30 PM	Blood test
	Insulin injection Regular (short-acting)
	Lunch
2:30 PM	Snack
	Blood test
4:30 PM	Snack
6:30 PM	Blood test
	Insulin injection Regular (short-acting)
	Dinner
8:30 PM	Blood test
	Insulin injection NPH (long-lasting)
	Snack

I work hard every day to balance what is going on in my body and to keep my blood sugars normal. Many things influence how insulin is absorbed and whether my blood sugar levels go up or down:

- **Exercise**: Lowers blood sugar rapidly. During soccer games, I snack every 15 minutes and do a blood sugar check at halftime.
- **Stress**: Usually lowers my blood sugar. During exams and heavy concentration, the brain absorbs enormous amounts of sugar. Blood sugar can drop dramatically causing lapses in mental function. I just can't think. Eating a snack and taking 5–10 minutes to absorb the glucose gets me back on track.
- **Cold**: Lowers blood sugar rapidly.
- **Heat**: Changes insulin needs.

- **Illness**: Usually causes a rise in blood sugar. When I am ill, I usually take two or three additional shots of Regular (short-acting insulin) per day, do frequent blood tests, and test for ketones.
- **Growth Spurts, Hormones**: Usually cause a rise in blood sugar, which can make you feel "hyper." Very high blood sugar usually causes sluggishness and an all-over sick feeling.

WHAT THE DOC SAYS:

Yet again, planning ahead, anticipating problems, and enlisting the understanding and support of the people around you is vitally important to provide the structure you need to truly be free and safe. There is nothing to be embarrassed about or ashamed of, so let all the adults or supervisors of your activities know your daily schedule. In fact, it can be a badge of pride to say, "I do everything I do in my life, **and** all this other stuff that most people don't have to!"

YOUR COOLER EQUALS FREEDOM

Once you get this routine down, you can do anything!

Keep a cooler at home, at school, and in each family car filled with:

- Short   Frosting, Gatorade, Cookies
- Medium   Cheez-Its
- Long   Jerky, Peanuts

Tip: Tape the **Symptoms** printout (page 104) in the top of every cooler. When the symptoms occur (when you are very low), one of your friends will know how to help you.

SUPPLIES TO KEEP AT HOME

■ **Always have these things on hand at home**. This makes life simpler and more routine. The sugar drinks and frosting you need for treating low blood sugar are not to be eaten by anybody else.

Frosting in a tub in the fridge	Gatorade	Orange juice
Frosting in tubes for emergencies	Crackers	Cookies
Real 7-Up and diet drinks	Jerky	Whole milk

All the kids in the family should know where the frosting is and should get it and give it to you immediately if you're feeling bad (1 big spoonful).

■ **Never put off eating when you have low blood sugar.** Follow frosting with whole milk. The sugar in the frosting will only last a few minutes. You'll need more long-lasting calories right away. Milk works great.

If these things are on hand at home, you can handle any situation. The frosting in the tub is for when you are really low and the same with the real 7-Up. Gatorade is good if you catch yourself crashing. Crackers and cookies are a good second snack, as is whole milk after a low blood sugar. Jerky just finishes off the snack, so you'll be in good shape.

Remember that we eat a snack every 2 hours.

WHAT THE DOC SAYS:

With newer rapid-acting insulin, many children and teenagers don't eat mid-morning snacks. It is important to determine your individual snack needs based on your insulin regimen and exercise programs.

18

Brothers and Sisters Speak

Diabetes has been a major part of my life and the rest of my family's since I was first diagnosed with it more than 15 years ago. We have all written various pieces about living with it either for school assignments or just to get our feelings out. My sister Mary wrote the following essay during her senior year at Nordhoff High School. She entered a statewide essay contest to answer the question, "Should animals be used in medical research?" She won a $500 scholarship for her essay. Even siblings who are not diabetics can benefit from putting their feelings down on paper. Mary has just graduated from medical school at USC.

My brother, Bo, made a picture book when he was six, just months after being diagnosed with diabetes himself. It was hard for him to write about himself, so he chose to write about me. Every kid with diabetes should write about how diabetes makes him or her feel. It helps a lot.

Kids, I'm Proud of You was written by our sister, Jenny. Jenny is the oldest and she was the boss when we were growing up. Don't let her 4′11″ stature fool you, Jenny is tough. She received her B.A. from Berkeley in 1996 and is currently the editor-in-chief of *Kitchen Sink*, a Bay-area culture and politics magazine. She is president of Neighbor Lady Community Art Project, a non-profit dedicated to arts and culture education.

The fourth piece is an email I wrote to Bo after my roommates at college had to call 911 for me. We figured out what happened and have included Spike's *911—One, Two, Three, Boom! You're Gone* to help you avoid the same situation. **This story is not for little kids.** When you go out on your own, you'll need to know how to handle every situation. We hope this will help.

WHY ANIMALS ARE USED IN BIOMEDICAL RESEARCH
by Mary Loy

The experimental use of animals in medical and biological sciences is something I consider not only a very important part of science, but it is also something that is important to me personally. My reasons for my avid support of scientific research on animals will be apparent when you read about a painful but sobering scenario that took place in my home less than a year ago.

"Mom, I'm hungry."

"I know, Honey, but you just ate."

"I'm so sick of this, Mom. I just want to be able to eat when I'm hungry like everybody else. Just give me a unit so I can eat."

A unit of insulin is what he meant. My brother is a diabetic. Diagnosed at age six, Thanksgiving day of 1988, exactly 1 year after my other brother had been diagnosed at age seven. Hearing these words come out of my baby brother's mouth, it hit me. I suddenly realized that he had been unjustly and cruelly stripped of his innocence. He was right—he was no longer "like everybody else."

When we are hungry, we eat; it's part of our nature. When we are tired, we sleep in. When we want to play, we play. But my brothers can't just spontaneously do these things. They have to worry about what and when they eat, how and when they exercise, and how much insulin they need each morning and night, every day of their lives.

I'm a practical person. When Spike got diabetes, it was a shock for the whole family, and it was an awful thing to have happen. But I decided that it was a part of all of our lives now, and we would just have to learn to deal with it however unpleasant or unfair it seemed. When Bodie turned up with it, and we hadn't found any traces of the disease anywhere in our family background, I thought that if there is a God, he must be mad at our family. I couldn't understand how such a freak thing could have happened to us. But again, I was determined not to get emotional. At least they were both still alive, I told myself. At least with modern technology, they would both be able to lead almost perfectly normal lives. Almost.

So when I heard my brother utter that pitiful plea, "Just give me a unit so I can eat" with tears in his eyes, I wanted to take him into my arms and assure him that everything was going to be all right. But I couldn't, because it wasn't. My little brother I saw as this little hellion running around without a worry in the world, and I always felt I could protect him and say, "Don't worry Bodie, I won't ever let anything bad happen to you." But he had been forced to grow up and become a responsible adult before most kids had learned to dress themselves. My image of him had changed; I no longer saw the same smiling, carefree kid. The smile was gone. I saw the eyes of an older man in my brother's eyes—one who had faced many hardships yet never found happiness.

Suddenly, all the problems I had considered to be such a big part of my life seemed insignificant and trivial. I was mad and frustrated. I couldn't protect little Bodie anymore; I couldn't undo what had already happened; I couldn't even take it away from him and put it in myself. I didn't want to be perfectly healthy while Bodie ("My little Prince" is what my mother always called him) had to suffer.

This thing, this disease has changed him, I thought. He's so much more responsible; he's even a bit more sensitive. But he shouldn't have to be.

I console myself now with the knowledge that research involving experiments with dogs and swine is being done right now to try to find a cure for diabetes. This research is so exciting to me because it may mean that my brothers will be cured in the not too distant future. Having seen some of the experiments involving swine first-hand, I have been so inspired that I plan my own future in the field of medical research.

So many people can benefit from what science discovers through the use of animals in research, and so many wonderful and brilliant discoveries have already been made. I have chosen to focus on only one reason that this area of science is so important simply because it is something that really hits home for me—and because I couldn't possibly cover everything that should be known about this marvelous field of study.

So when the question is asked, "Why are animals used in biomedical research?" My answer is, "Because of my brothers and others like them who can benefit from such research." If it can make a little boy's tears go away, nothing is more important.

KIDS, I'M PROUD OF YOU
by Jenny Loy

When Spike got diabetes, we all learned about how to be patient and help him when he was low and how to give shots.

Even baby Bo, who was only 5 years old, knew where the frosting was and walked around the house practicing injecting an orange. Then Bo got diabetes, and we were really busy.

Mom was proud of us. "Kids, I'm proud of you, all of you." That's what she said one afternoon, herding us into the living room from the far corners of our after-school lives. Spike and Bo shuffled their feet a bit and the dirt from their latest war games sifted audibly to the floor. Mary and I stood behind the boys poking at them to watch the dust cloud slowly engulf their feet.

"Listen you guys, I'm really pleased with the way you've all worked together. You are like a little army taking care of each other. You've all been so wonderful." (You know how moms get.) "Your dad and I think you deserve a reward."

"Like what? A pack of gum?" I asked.

"No, a big reward," she came back. "You guys think of something you would really like to do, something big."

A huddle just wasn't going to be sufficient. Mary grabbed Bodie by the hand and I yanked Spike's collar. We hustled out of the living room so fast that the boys' GI Joe dust cloud was all that was left to hear Mom's hints. "You all like the ocean," she prattled away, "I was thinking of a trip to Hawaii this summer. I want to do something special for all of you."

We corralled the boys in the hallway where we could converse with, cajole, and possibly torture our younger siblings into agreeing with what we, the older sisters who obviously knew best, decided what the "kids" wanted.

Twenty minutes later, returning to the living room, the four angels she was so proud of just a moment before announced to Mom that we had unanimously decided that we wanted to be in the movies! (Well, I announced it because it really was my idea. I'm the kid that was born to be a star.)

I can tell you she was surprised. "You're sure you don't want to go to Hawaii?"

"No, we want to be in the movies. Movies, movies," Bodie chanted.

That afternoon began yet another chapter in the lives of the Loy children. She did it. She gave us our reward. We had head shots taken by a professional photographer, and we signed up with an agent. For the next 3 years, Mom drove each of us down to LA as we were called to be extras. Our favorite job by far was the day we got paid to ride the roller coaster at Magic Mountain. After a few rides, one by one, the adult extras they had hired to make a Mylanta commercial started climbing out of the roller coaster. There they were, lying on the platform, holding their stomachs and moaning. Pretty soon it was just us four kids and Mom, riding the Colossus over and over. They shot the scene 33 times, then sent us over to The Revolution. I think we rode The Revolution about a dozen times. What a great day!

Mary and I stopped doing extra work when we got into high school. Spike and Bo held out until their acting careers threatened to interfere with baseball practice.

911—ONE, TWO, THREE, BOOM! YOU'RE GONE

After Spike had been away at college for a few months, he got really sick with the flu and his roommate had to call 911. This is the first time a super low blood sugar has ever happened to either of us. We put this in our book because maybe by understanding what happened to Spike, you can avoid ever getting this low. And, don't get scared, everything turned out all right! Here is his email.

Subj: low
Date: 2/5/99 9:24:48 AM Pacific Standard Time
From: Spike@stanford.edu
To: Bo

Had a rough day of snowboarding in some butt cold weather. Ate at Kentucky Fried Chicken on the way home. I ate a lot and took only ⅔ of my normal dose of insulin. The drive home from Tahoe was uneventful.

Then I get home and start feeling a little queasy and/or low. I test my blood sugar and I am about 70 (that's just the slightest bit low). So I decide I had better eat a little to bring my sugar back up. I eat, but soon after I throw up quite a bit. This has happened before and I know that after throwing up I need to eat to replenish my sugars, so I eat and drink some more. I throw up a bunch again. I am feeling pretty bad at this point, pretty sick, and a little low, and really tired. I eat some more and lie down on my bed.

I wake up two hours later with five paramedics in my room, the residential fellow, two residential advisors and about four of my friends. But the cool stuff happened when I was unconscious and coming to.

Brad, my roommate tells me that while lying in bed, I made a kind of gurgled mutter and fell out of bed (luckily I had just lowered my bed the week before). He kicked me or did something to try to rouse me, but I would have none of it, so he went and got Danny (our friend in the room across the hall). Danny couldn't wake me up and neither could Luke. So they called 911. The paramedics got there in 2 minutes flat (pretty good response time if you ask me—pretty reassuring).

Meanwhile, inside my head it felt like I was spinning. Each second or so I would see a new person in my room who was doing something new to me. The rate at which the strangers were flashing on the scene and bugging me started accelerating. I was spinning faster and faster, seeing someone new more and more rapidly and becoming more and more annoyed. Pretty psychedelic.

I remember thinking to myself, OK, Spike, this is just some dream. To make all these guys go away, so I can get some sleep, I just need to block them all out at once. I tried blocking them out. That didn't work. OK, then, I said to myself, I need to make them go away one by one.

I stood up, stared at one of the people in my room and said, "One, two, three, Boom! You're gone!" Then I looked through someone else and said, "One, two, three, Boom! You're gone!" After one, two, three, booming them away for a little while, the paramedics made me sit down, and shot me up with some glucagon. (That's an insulin inhibitor that gets the sugar to the brain faster.)

"Spike, can you hear me?"

"Who are you?"

"I'm Chris. I'm a paramedic. Can you hear me?"

"Yes."

"What day is it?"

"Ummm, Sunday night or Monday morning."

"Sure is."

I let out a sigh of relief. "Give me 3 seconds." I closed my eyes and counted, "One, two, three." I didn't say "Boom! You're gone" this time; I just opened my eyes and said, "Wow! You're still here."

"Spike, can you tell me who your friends are?"

"Sure." I looked around. "There's Luke. Brad's here, and Danny of course. Damn!"

The paramedics asked if I wanted to be hospitalized, and at first I said, yes, but pretty soon I was fully back to normal (as normal as I am ever gonna get) and told him I was fine (which I was). I asked Chris what my sugar was and he told me that when they first got there I was 39 (pretty low) but that it had risen to 370 or so (pretty high).

The paramedics all left and my friends stuck around and made fun of me for a while, each one in turn imitating my "One, two, three, Boom! You're gone" routine. What good friends I've met here. Not only do they save my life, but they stick around to laugh about it. Golly.

Looking back on this, we know it happened because of a combination of things.

1. Spike took too much insulin. Spike had been exercising all day. He took 10 units of Regular (short acting) insulin at dinner, not his usual 15, but that was still too much. He should have taken only 5 or 6 units.
2. He threw up. Remember the section, When You Are Sick on page 73? Vomiting calls for special action.
   Throw up once: call someone.
   Throw up twice: call the doctor, or get help.
3. His friends didn't know about glucagon. They do now! They did the right thing by calling 911, but they could have tried injecting Spike with glucagon when he wouldn't wake up. That would probably have been all that he needed.

We have written up a protocol for when you are sick: It's taped on Spike's closet door right now. You may want to hang it up on yours, too.

PROTOCOL FOR WHEN YOU ARE SICK

Throw up once: Tell a friend. Don't be alone. Call home so they can check on you for the next few hours.

Throw up twice: Go to the clinic at school. **Don't go alone.**

Glucagon: Have your glucagon kit in your fridge.

Instructions: Tape glucagon instructions on your closet door.

911: Go ahead and call 911 if things get out of hand.

GLUCAGON INSTRUCTIONS

Glucagon isn't just sugar as the name sounds. It is an anti-insulin hormone. That's why even when you can't eat any food, an injection of glucagon will raise your blood sugar immediately.

When Do You Use Glucagon?

Inject Spike with glucagon if you can't wake him up or if he is so disoriented he doesn't make sense and you can't get him to eat.

How Do You Use Glucagon?

1. Inject the liquid in the syringe into the bottle of glucagon powder.
2. Shake the bottle until the glucagon dissolves and becomes clear.
3. Draw all the glucagon solution into the syringe. (For kids under 45 lbs. use ½.)
4. Inject all the solution into the leg or butt.
5. Put Spike on his side, because when he wakes up, he may throw up.

6. Give food as soon as he wakes up: Gatorade, crackers, cookies, or anything he can eat.

Keep glucagon in your fridge.
Always take your glucagon kit on trips.

Note: I had a second episode of falling blood sugars and the flu in February, 2001. I called home for support and gave myself a glucagon injection. (My roommate could have done it, but I wanted to.) Within minutes my sugar was up and the low blood sugar episode passed. Don't be scared if you have to use glucagon. It works, and it won't hurt you.

19

Tips

LOW BLOOD SUGAR

When you have a low blood sugar, eat first, test later.

ALWAYS HAVE FOOD

Always carry a granola bar in your pocket in case you get low.

CAR RIDES

Always have a packed cooler in any car you ride in. If you forget it, go back for it.

MONEY

You need a few dollars with you at all times in case you need to buy food.

FROSTING

We carry Cake Mate decorating gel—the 99-cent tube. It works when we're low.

GLUCAGON

Take a glucagon kit when you are traveling, camping, or back-packing.

6-WEEK RULE

Throw away opened insulin after 6 weeks because it loses its potency.

AT RESTAURANTS

At restaurants order food first. When it reaches the table, then shoot up.

TWO OF EVERYTHING

Have two of everything at home—insulin, finger prick devices, batteries, Inject-ease. Things break.

DOUBLE UP

Take two sets of insulin on trips. Sometimes the glass bottles break. Keep insulin with you. It can freeze in the luggage compartment or go bad when it gets too hot. Take an extra battery for your glucose meter.

TRAVELING

When we travel, we each carry backpacks containing our insulin kit, record book, Gatorade, frosting, crackers, cookies, and jerky. Have your mom or dad carry a third back-up backpack, packed with the same things.

HOSPITALS

If you are going to the hospital, for example for surgery, take your kit!

WATER SPORTS

Put a Cake Mate frosting in your wetsuit.

COMFORT

Try an Inject-ease. We found that it makes life easier. (An Inject-ease is a device that puts the needle into the skin so you don't have to.)

WHERE TO PRICK

Don't prick the tips of your fingers; prick the sides of the finger pad—it feels better. With some new meters, you can prick your forearm. Be sure to rub your arm before pricking, so you'll get enough blood. Bo says they don't hurt.

WHERE TO INJECT

My favorite place is the top of the hip. I sometimes do it in the arm and the leg.

CHEMSTRIPS

If you're using blood sugar test strips that can be read by eye, you can cut them in half.

STORING USED SYRINGES

Spike and I keep our syringes in 5-gallon water bottles. When we are done with the syringes, we put the orange top back on but not the bottom white part because that makes it look like an unused syringe. Pharmacies also carry Sharps containers that you can use. At a friend's house, you can put the orange top back on your used syringes and then put them in an empty soda bottle or just keep them in your kit to take back home.

TELL EVERYONE YOU KNOW THAT YOU HAVE DIABETES

You need to do this so friends and grown-ups can help you when you are low and so they can get involved.

BE SAFE

When you go to school, go surfing, go to practice, go to a friend's, go in a car, or go anywhere, carry your backpack or a cooler. Then you are safe, and no one has to worry.

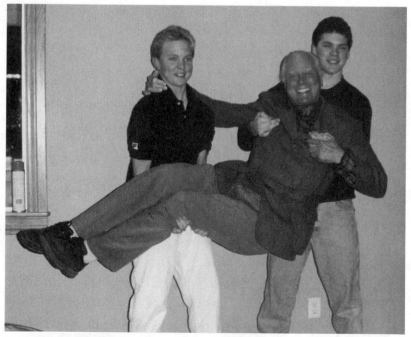

Bo and Spike, lending friend Larry Hagman a hand

20

The Family Scrapbook

We cannot stress enough how beneficial getting involved with research is. It gives us a great sense of hope. It also leads to a much greater understanding of what is going on with your condition. We have an ongoing scrapbook of our involvement, and it won't be finished until we can add the hospital papers documenting our successful islet cell transplants or the receipt from a closed loop continuous monitor/pump system.

We met Dr. Patrick Soon-Shiong at the UCLA Transplant Lab. He told us how difficult it was to find pigs for research and asked for our help. Since we live on a small ranch, we were able to raise a special breed of pigs, Great Whites, for research. Great Whites have pancreatic cells that may some-day be transplanted into humans. We raised them, slaughtered them, and my mother surgically removed their pancreases and transported them to Dr. Patrick Soon-Shiong's lab. Bo was six and I was eight years old when we started doing this, so our job was to be the timers. We timed how long it took to remove the pancreas and get it safely in the preservation solution. Bo sometimes actually put on surgical gloves and helped

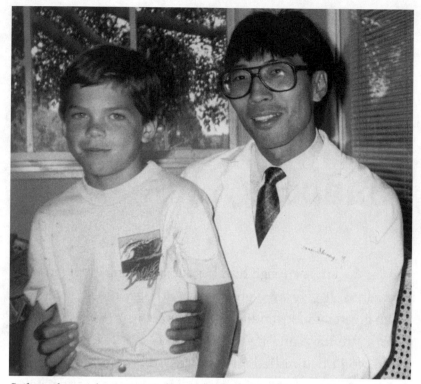

Spike and transplant research doctor, Patrick Soon-Shiong, 1987

with the pancreas removal. We didn't have huge amounts of money to donate, but we did have space to raise these animals and time to do the weekly surgeries, so we did it. (We shared the meat with neighbors, so nothing was wasted.)

Being actively involved with the research gives me more hope for the future than anything else, and it has sparked my interest in entering the field of diabetes research as a profession after college.

GET EXCITED ABOUT RESEARCH

Since we were diagnosed with diabetes, our family has been actively involved in diabetes research. There are currently many fields of research ranging from looking for the cure to research into technologies to make our lives even easier and make diabetes even less of a nuisance.

Major fields of research are:

Islet Transplants

Transplanting human and pig islet cells encapsulated in a semi-permeable membrane to protect them from the immune system, which would eliminate the need for daily injections. (This is the field we were working on with Dr. Soon Shiong.)

Glucose Monitoring

Development of new ways to monitor your blood sugar without having so many finger pricks, including the Glucowatch and implantable devices to give continuous monitoring.

The GlucoWatch Biographer

Non-invasive glucose monitoring for adults, gives 3 readings an hour for 12 hours.

Genetic Engineering

Creating better forms of human insulin.

Insulin Pumps

Development of improved, smarter insulin pumps to replace daily injections.

Nasal Sprays and Pills

This method of insulin administration is in the trial stages.

Inhalator

Creating an oral insulin delivery sysem.

Vaccine

Screening of high-risk individuals who have family histories of diabetes and finding ways to prevent the immune system from destroying islet cells.

There are hundreds of labs investigating diabetes around the country and around the globe. Donating money, time, or resources makes you feel like you are actually a part of the quest for the cure that is so close. Wouldn't it be great to be able to say "I was a part of this" on the day that you get your cure?

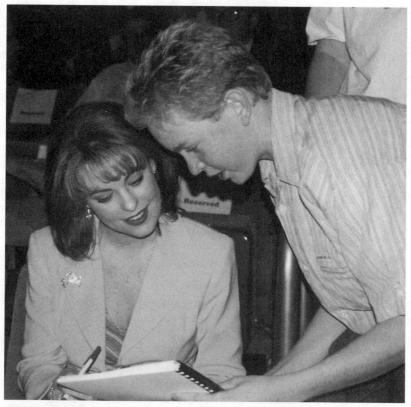

Bo and Nicole Johnson, Miss America 1999

Other Books to Read

If you would like to learn more about diabetes, here are books we recommend. All are available at bookstores, Amazon.com, and store.diabetes.org. (Contact us at boandspike@aol.com)

487 Really Cool Tips for Kids with Diabetes by us and about 114 other kids.

Real Life Parenting of Kids With Diabetes by Virginia Nasmyth Loy. This is a companion book to *Getting a Grip*. Our book, *Getting a Grip* is a how-to book for kids and teens. *Real Life Parenting* is the how-to book for parents, teachers, coaches and friends. *Real Life Parenting* includes a large section on toddlers and a chapter on going off to college!

The Schwarzbein Principle by Diana Schwarzbein, MD. Dr. Diana is our endocrinologist. Meeting her changed our lives. Your parents should read this entire book. It makes sense of what is going on in your body on a cellular level. Everything about food, calories, sugar, and carbohydrates turning into sugar is explained. We use *The Schwarzbein Principle* to balance our diet. This book is available from Amazon.com and bookstores everywhere.

A Field Guide to Type 1 Diabetes by ADA. A good exploration of diabetes and how to live with it.

Smart Pumping for People with Diabetes by Howard Walpert, MD. Everything you'll need to know about insulin pumps by a Joslin Center pump master.

An Instructional Aid on Juvenile Diabetes Mellitus by Luther B. Travis, MD. This book is available from Amazon.com and bookstores everywhere.

Taking Diabetes to School by Kim Grossalin et al. This is a good book for grade school kids to share with their teachers and fellow students. Available through Amazon.com.

The Dinosaur Tamer by Marcia Levine Mazur, Peter Banks, and Andrew Keegan. A collection of 25 stories for kids with diabetes from *Diabetes Forecast* Kid's Corner.

Getting the Most Out of Diabetes Camp: A Guidebook for Parents and Kids by ADA.

Cooking Up Fun for Kids with Diabetes by Patti B. Geil, MS, RD, COE, and Tami A. Ross, RD, CDE. Have fun creating diabetes friendly, cool kids' foods.

Index

About the American Diabetes Association

The American Diabetes Association is the nation's leading voluntary health organization supporting diabetes research, information, and advocacy. Its mission is to prevent and cure diabetes and to improve the lives of all people affected by diabetes. The American Diabetes Association is the leading publisher of comprehensive diabetes information. Its huge library of practical and authoritative books for people with diabetes covers every aspect of self-care—cooking and nutrition, fitness, weight control, medications, complications, emotional issues, and general self-care.

To order American Diabetes Association books: Call 1-800-232-6733. http://store.diabetes.org [Note: there is no need to use **www** when typing this particular Web address]

To join the American Diabetes Association: Call 1-800-806-7801. www.diabetes.org/membership

For more information about diabetes or ADA programs and services: Call 1-800-342-2383). E-mail: Customerservice@diabetes.org www.diabetes.org

To locate an ADA/NCQA Recognized Provider of quality diabetes care in your area: www.ncqa.org/dprp

To find an ADA Recognized Education Program in your area: Call 1-888-232-0822. www.diabetes.org/recognition/education.asp

To join the fight to increase funding for diabetes research, end discrimination, and improve insurance coverage: Call 1-800-342-2383. www.diabetes.org /advocacy

To find out how you can get involved with the programs in your community: Call 1-800-342-2383). See below for program Web addresses.

- *American Diabetes Month:* educational activities aimed at those diagnosed with diabetes—month of November. www.diabetes.org/ADM
- *American Diabetes Alert:* annual public awareness campaign to find the undiagnosed—held the fourth Tuesday in March. www.diabetes.org/alert
- *The Diabetes Assistance & Resources Program (DAR):* diabetes awareness program targeted to the Latino community. www.diabetes.org/DAR
- *African American Program:* diabetes awareness program targeted to the African American community. www.diabetes.org/africanamerican
- *Awakening the Spirit: Pathways to Diabetes Prevention & Control:* diabetes awareness program targeted to the Native American community. www.diabetes.org/awakening

To find out about an important research project regarding type 2 diabetes: www.diabetes.org/ada/research.asp

To obtain information on making a planned gift or charitable bequest: Call 1-888-700-7029. www.diabetes.org/ada/plan.asp

To make a donation or memorial contribution: Call 1-800-342-2383. www.diabetes.org/ada/cont.asp